A NEW YOU

USING THE BODY'S REGENERATIVE AND RESTORATIVE HEALING POWERS to OPTIMIZE ORTHOPEDIC, HORMONAL and SEXUAL HEALTH FUNCTION

MICHAEL J. MEIGHEN, MD
#1 Bestselling Author

Learn more about Dr. Meighen at
www.EmpoweredWellnessNC.com

A NEW YOU
USING THE BODY'S REGENERATIVE AND RESTORATIVE
HEALING POWERS TO OPTIMIZE ORTHOPEDIC, HORMONAL
AND SEXUAL HEALTH FUNCTION

Description: First edition | August 2018
ISBN 9781719880664 (paperback) |

Limit of Liability/Disclaimer of Warranty

While the author has used their best efforts in preparing this
report, they make no representation or warranties with
respect to the accuracy or completeness of the contents and
specifically disclaim any implied warranties. The advice and
strategies contained herein may not be suitable for your
situation. You should consult with a professional where
appropriate. The author shall not be liable for any loss of
profit or any other commercial damages, including but not
limited to special, incidental, consequential or other damages.

Table of Contents

CHAPTER 1: MY STORY

My journey and transformation like most people started at a very young age. There were a few events that shaped my youth into young adulthood. The first event was the divorce of my parents at the age of 11. This was incredibly difficult as my parents were still quite young (in their early 30's) and I had twin 8-year old brothers. This placed a significant amount of responsibility on my shoulders to care for them as a surrogate parent, but also navigate the tense relationship that was my parents. This development forced me to abandon my childhood and shoulder more of the load in relation to life and daily activities. On a positive note, I became adept at organization, cooking, cleaning, laundry, and time management. I also learned to manage the multiple needs of people and their personalities allowing me to become more versatile and adapted in relation to assessment and management techniques. My major escape during these times was my love of athletics and competition. This topic will become an eternal theme on my life as you will see throughout the forthcoming pages of this book.

The second occurrence that considerably changed my life and pushed me towards a career in medicine was in fact a tragedy. I was playing football in 8th grade as a tight end. I went out for a pass and got hit from the side and fractured my right tibia and fibula. The pain was tremendous and really brought tears to my eyes. I knew I was done for the season, and it ultimately ended my football career. I was placed into a cast for eight weeks at the beginning of the school year. I felt like a ghost in relation to my interaction with my teammates and my school friends. I felt as though I was on an island and isolated from many of the activities that I had been involved with just days or weeks before the trauma.

This however provided me with an opportunity to interact with orthopedic surgeons, physical therapists, and other sports medicine professionals. This laid the foundation for my career in orthopedic medicine and fitness. I had always been interested in science from an early age including biology, chemistry, and human performance. I was uncertain as to my direction, but this negative turned into a positive as it provided a focus for my future.

I healed after eight weeks and started a physical therapy and home exercise regimen. I eventually returned to basketball that fall and completed the season without incident. I was getting ready for baseball in the spring when I received some devastating news. In a routine follow-up with my orthopedic surgeon Dr. Thompson, x-rays and clinical exam showed that I had injured my growth plate with the fracture and my leg was growing at an angle. Since I had multiple years left to grow, I would need to have two surgeries. The first was to treat the left leg with an osteotomy to remove bone and kill the growth plate so this side would stop growing such that the legs would not be two different lengths. The second was to cut the bone on the right and straighten the leg to restore length and kill the growth plate from the knee down. To say the least, I was devastated. I would basically be in and out of hospitals over the next 6 months and embark on a long recovery with therapy and home exercise. I now joke that the fracture and two surgeries ended my NBA career. These events allowed me the opportunity to struggle and fight my way through adversity. It also allowed me to become a patient and thus understand the difficulty and struggle of receiving bad news; and how this may affect a person from a physical, mental, emotional, and overall health standpoint.

I fully recovered from the surgeries and competed in multiple sports in high school including baseball, basketball,

and golf. I was also able to play multiple intramural and club
sports in college without incident. It also fueled my passion
for exercise including strength training, aerobic fitness,
flexibility training, nutrition, and human performance. The
energy for these activities and the quest for knowledge on
these topics persists even today. I have in fact signed on to a
program taught by fitness guru Ben Greenfield to further my
education and receive certification through KionU to further
enhance my ability to treat patients and teach clients. Fitness
in my opinion is the cornerstone of health and the starting
point for all musculoskeletal treatments and health
transformations. I will expound upon this topic in other
areas in the book. The human body was made for movement
and activity. We have lost this focus along the way with
modern conveniences which have made us sedentary and
lazy. Poor diet and nutrition, stress, pharmaceuticals,
environmental toxins, and sleep issues have also negatively
affected health and left us with an obesity crisis. The country
and the world need to target the current and future healthcare
emergency; otherwise, this issue will devastate generations
moving forward.

CHAPTER 2: CROSSROADS

A great song and live album by Eric Clapton or a bad movie with Ralph Macchio of Karate Kid fame.

I feel in many ways that my life, my career, and my future had reached a crossroads. This crisis feeling had been slowly building for the last 5-10 years. I had been involved in healthcare for 23+ years primarily in the orthopedic and outpatient musculoskeletal realm. I was seeing and treating 100-150 patients a week and making more money than I ever dreamed possible. I however was miserable, depressed, and despondent. There were a few reasons for these feelings.

The first was that while I was seeing and treating a number of people with various tools such as medication, physical therapy, injections, rest, and surgery; very few (less than 10%) of the patients were improving to the satisfaction of either myself or the patient. The limited time spent with the patient barely scratched the surface of identifying the true cause for their symptoms and ultimately limited their response. The treatments themselves were also ineffective because they failed to heal and restore the patient. They primarily covered or masked symptoms and failed to impact health in a positive manner.

The second was goals of the clinic failed to align with my belief system. I wanted to use any tool available including regenerative medicine procedures, hormone replacement, functional medicine, psychological medicine, personal training, and personalized treatment plans to transform the patient in hopes of healing them for both the present and the future. I also wanted patients to avoid surgery and medications and focus on non-operative and total body health optimization. This model would have been a blend of insurance and cash-based options. The goals of the group were more focused on imaging studies, procedures, surgeries, and drugs. The things that would make money but not necessarily improve health quality. Creative and out of the box thinking was frowned upon due to a number of concerns. These included diminishing the number of surgical procedures, scope of practice questions, lawsuit concerns, a limited understanding of the literature, and poor vetting of patient needs and wants.

I will provide a few examples. I had a partner, Dr. Total Joint (not his real name to protect the innocent) whom needed some help. The total joint patients that he was seeing needed to make some positive changes in their life in order to undergo either total hip or total knee joint procedures. This started as the result of bundled payments where the insurance provider would pay a flat fee to cover all required services of the procedure. The less complications that occurred improved the reimbursement for all of those involved. The more complications reduced the payment and ultimately penalized the involved providers and healthcare facilities. Dr. Total Joint had a number of patients whom had an elevated BMI (body mass index), diabetes mellitus and elevated hemoglobin A1C (a measure of blood sugars over a 60-90 day period), and anemia. These abnormalities placed the patient in a higher risk category which tended to increase the complication rate and the cost. He therefore needed help with improving these parameters as he was getting limited help from the primary care doctors due to our sick care system. We have the great ability to Maintain Disease and therefore a perfect acronym for MD in our current regimen. We however have a poor understanding of preventative and restorative measures to help with chronic health issues like weight loss, diabetes, anemia, hypercholesterolemia, and osteoporosis. Dr. Total Joint knew that I had been training in hormone replacement and functional medicine and therefore he sent me some of his folks to try to remedy their issues such that they he could treat their joint problems. To make a long story short (topics I will expound upon later in the book), we were successful in improving the parameters for the four patients that he sent to me for treatment. I was also able to improve the bone health of these patients further limiting the complication rate. Everybody was happy: myself, the patients, Dr. Total Joint, the clinic, the hospital, etc. I therefore felt that this was a project that deserved further exploration and a potential treatment plan that could be reproduced clinic wide. This would improve patient and physician satisfaction and limit referrals outside of the clinic. This was also an area of interest and a passion of mine to help people transform their lives. I therefore presented the plan with a focus on weight loss, osteoporosis, and regenerative medicine with a goal of opening a separate center. I felt that the presentation went well and I was really excited about the possibilities for a positive change in my career path. The group however failed to share my excitement in this creative endeavor. They failed to endorse the project and in fact told me that I had to discontinue all hormone and functional medicine treatments due to fear and concerns about scope of practice. I was disappointed and devastated which served to negate my ingenuity and pushed me further into a state of depression. I was also angry that I had to stop treatment on patients that were benefitting from the therapy and were actually happy that somebody had actually listened to them and addressed their life limiting issues like fatigue, pain, and sexual dysfunction. This setback only fueled my desire to find a better way.

The second occurrence involved a medical colleague I had seen for shoulder pain. His workup showed him to have both a rotator cuff tear and a labral tear. Surgery was recommended by one of my partners. In retrospect, I wish at the time I would have had the capability to inject him with stem cells as I feel as though his outcome would have been outstanding, but I digress. Prior to the procedure, we discussed his case in detail and we both mutually theorized that maximizing his testosterone and growth hormone may have a positive effect on his recovery and outcome. He therefore maximized both levels with the help of his partner. The surgery went off without a hitch. Pain medicine needs lasted only 2-3 days. The rehabilitation program progressed well and ahead of schedule. Again, everybody involved was happy with the outcome. This case was presented to the group including the research department as a potential study to assess outcome improvement from rotator cuff repair with hormone optimization. This also went over like a lead balloon and gained little to no traction. Ideas squashed and hopes dashed but I was not deterred.

The final issue was the lack of initiative by the patients themselves and the fact that many had no goals in mind as they presented to see me for treatment. It was not uncommon for a patient to respond, "I don't know" or "my doctor sent me" when they were asked why they were in the office. Others had an agenda to avoid something and wanted documentation and justification for their actions. These things included work excuses, jury duty waivers, disability forms, travel insurance cancellations, and gym membership discontinuations. I was also shocked and surprised at the number of folks that totally resisted the recommendations for exercise, physical therapy, and personal training. In my opinion, exercise and fitness are the 1st line and most cost-effective interventions that healthcare providers can prescribe. Yet, people were more interested in drugs including pain pills (opioids) and anxiety medicines (benzodiazepines). Neither of these drug groups have been shown to be helpful or effective for long term management of pain problems or psychological problems in any evidence-based studies. They in fact cause significant harm including addiction, hormone dysregulation, and sudden death. I was also surprised at the number of patients that felt that one injection either into a joint or into their spine would be the cure all for the years of neglect and abuse. The vast majority of people took better care of their pets and their cars than themselves. They were also in denial in relation to the affect that their chronic health issues were having on their orthopedic problems and functional deficits. People continuously showed poor insight into their limitations and the effect it was having on them today, but also how it would affect them in the future. Due to time constraints, I was unable to educate them on the number of issues that were affecting them and oftentimes the musculoskeletal problem was lower down on the totem pole of their problems. The vast majority of patients were obese, deconditioned, depressed, anxious, tired, and overmedicated. These diverse set of problems in my opinion needed to be addressed prior to treating their knee or their spine. Otherwise, the outcomes were sure to suffer along with patient and physician satisfaction. I however typically had 15-20 minutes and limited resources to handle the overall patient which caused a significant amount of frustration and hand-wringing. Nobody was benefitting from this current patient care model.

CHAPTER 3: THE EPIPHANY

As my medical career evolved, I was learning more things from courses that I attended. Injection procedures for headache, spine pain, joint pain, soft tissue pain, and nerve pain. These oftentimes improved symptoms in the short term, but not in the long term. These procedures primarily consisted of using an injectable steroid which had the capability of calming inflammation but failed to heal or improve the underlying issue or problem. Inflammation gets a bad rap from both the medical literature and lay press, but it is imperative for healing injury and restoring function. When we use these injection procedures with steroid, we halt the progression of healing and cause more degradation, necrosis, and cell death. This has negative effects on the following structures: joints causing cartilage and stem cell death encouraging osteoarthritis, soft tissues causing ligament laxity and joint instability, tendons causing tears and functional weakness, and discs causing degeneration and herniation. All of these things would be termed a poor outcome and cause undo pain and harm to the individual patient. This did not seem to be the proper path to follow for short and long-term management of these problems.

We were also taught to employ and prescribe a number of drugs for these abnormalities in hopes of improving the symptoms including the pain and dysfunction. Oftentimes, these agents caused more side effect issues and problems which were more of an issue than the injury or disease. I will provide two examples. The first are anti-inflammatory drugs for pain like Motrin and Naprosyn. We were taught that these medications were first line therapy for acute and chronic musculoskeletal pain problems. There are a few problems however with this line of thinking. Similar to the aforementioned issues with steroids, anti-inflammatories block inflammation and halt the healing process necessary for recovery. They can also cause a gastrointestinal bleed which can be both costly for the system and life threatening for the patient. The second is the use of seizure medications like Neurontin for nerve or neuropathic pain. These medications are sedating and for that reason poorly tolerated. They also have a profound effect on balance leading to falls and subsequent fractures. This again seemed like poor form and not the ideal and proper way to manage patients. Our Hippocratic Oath tells us "To Do No Harm." Unfortunately, this was exactly what we were doing.

Something needed to change, and in a hurry, as I was churning through patients but helping very few of them to improve, recover, succeed, and prosper. I attended a meeting hosted by the American Academy of Orthopedic Medicine (AAOM) in 2005. This group of eclectic healthcare providers focus on treatment options that would be considered fringe or cutting edge. The meeting focus was on prolotherapy. This is an injection therapy using dextrose to help regenerate tendon, ligaments, soft tissues and restore stability to a joint. This treatment actually promotes inflammation via injection of the fluid which causes local trauma and recruits growth factors and fibroblasts (cells that release proteins critical for healing). As we have seen in other parts of the book, acute inflammation is imperative for healing of all injuries and limiting the negative effects of instability. This was truly one of the first regenerative therapies which started in the 1950s and was popularized by Dr. George Hackett, Dr. Earl Gedney, and Dr. James Cyriax. The teaching faculty at the meeting had similar issues and concerns with the so-called standard of care using steroid injections and medications. They were singing the praises of this intervention and its utility in healing. This treatment however was not well accepted by the general medical community and was criticized soundly as useless due to the limited number of studies on the process. I concur that the data on the subject was limited and scant at the time, but that does not mean that the treatment has no value. It just required further study. The data since that time has shown positive results in double blinded studies as compared to placebo and steroid treatments.

I now had a tool that seemed to fit well with my mindset and way of thinking. A low risk option with a medication in dextrose that has essentially no side effects and no systemic issues. The procedure provided great utility as it could be used for muscle, tendon, ligament, nerve and joint issues. It could be performed via palpation or with image guidance including ultrasound and fluoroscopy. There also were no limits on the number of injections that could be performed. All things were looking positive, but there were some drawbacks. This was considered an experimental procedure and therefore not covered by insurance. Thus, the procedure would be paid out of pocket. Our malpractice carrier at the time was also questioning the validity of covering it due to its experimental nature, but they eventually relented and covered it. My interest was piqued and my treatment armamentarium was now growing in a positive and helpful direction for my patients.

CHAPTER 4: REGENERATIVE MEDICINE PART I - PROLOTHERAPY

I returned to my clinic and soon began to search for appropriate candidates for this new intervention. There were a number of potential candidates with muscle, soft tissue, tendon, ligament, and joint issues. There was initially some hesitancy from patients in moving forward with the procedure due to the fact that it was not covered by any commercial insurance, and thus a personal cost to them. This fact allowed me to educate the patients on the procedure and the main positive that it was potentially healing as opposed to palliative. I also discussed the fact that no prior approvals would be necessary and that no denials would be made by an insurance carrier which can be particularly frustrating to all involved. The other important factor involved was the lack of response that the patients received from other conventional treatments. Things like medications, steroid injections, physical therapy, chiropractic, surgery and the like failed to improve their symptoms to the point that they were looking for alternatives. Therefore, there were candidates whom decided to take the plunge and move forward with the treatment. I will provide an example to illustrate this point.

Joe Hipp (not his real name) was a 75-year old male whom presented to my clinic one day with right lateral hip pain. The patient's symptoms had been ongoing for about 12-18 months. The symptoms started without a specific injury or trauma and was starting to limit his mobility and exercise tolerance. He was also starting to notice issues with walking, climbing, and squatting. He had been seen by his primary MD and started on Naprosyn (NSAID) and Ultram (pain reliever). This provided him limited benefit and therefore he sought the help of an orthopedic surgeon. He had x-rays performed which were normal and was ultimately diagnosed with trochanteric bursitis. He received a cortisone injection without imaging and was started in physical therapy. The injection provided him a few days' worth of benefit and the therapy helped minimally. Delving deeper however into his therapy treatment, I found that he was primarily treated with modalities and no strength training. This is a major pet peeve of mine which will be discussed further in the exercise and strength training chapters. Needless to say, functional strength training must be an integral part of an exercise routine otherwise the outcome will be poor. The patient had also received chiropractic and massage with minimal relief.

Mr. Hipp was frustrated with his pain, impairment, and limitation. He was no longer exercising regularly and he had subsequently gained about 20 lbs. He had also discontinued fishing which was one of his main hobbies due to the discomfort and concerns of falling getting into and out of the boat. He was down about his problems and noted feeling depressed. On exam, the patient had a noticeable limp on the right side. He had difficulty standing on his right leg and performing a single leg step-up on the right. He had palpable tenderness over the lateral hip toward the bony prominence called the greater trochanter which becomes evident if you push your hip out laterally. He was also very weak in his right lateral hip and buttock muscles. I believed that the patient had a gluteal tendon tear which was the cause of his weakness, pain, and dysfunction. Gluteal tendon issues are more common than previously believed and the diagnosis of trochanteric bursitis is typically over diagnosed. This has been documented in multiple studies in patients with hip pain that were imaged with MRI. I therefore ordered an MRI of his hip which confirmed a partial thickness gluteus medius tear with some atrophy (shrinkage) of his gluteal muscles. This confirmed my suspicion, and we therefore discussed prolotherapy injections. I discussed that it would typically take 3-6 procedures performed every month or so to help with this type problem. I discussed the fact that we would use both x-ray and ultrasound guidance for the injection. I also noted that the needle would be used in a pecking manner to cause microtrauma and encourage blood flow which helps with healing via a platelet response. The patient would also be started in an appropriate therapy program encouraging function and strength training. Mr. Hipp received 4 total injections which improved his pain by 80-90%. His gait issues normalized and his strength returned to normal. He was able to resume exercise which improved his weight and his overall mood. He returned to fishing which made both the patient and his wife happy as he was able to get out of the house and improve his disposition. The patient was pleased with his outcome and his new-found lease on life. I have had many similar responses with other patients as well. I was encouraged and excited, but I felt that there was more to be explored and learned.

CHAPTER 5: REGENERATIVE MEDICINE PART II - PLATELET RICH PLASMA (PRP)

The next part of the puzzle for restorative medicine and health optimization was the advent of injecting platelets. The procedure became popularized in the 1990s by plastic surgeons to help with wound healing and dentists to help with dry sockets and temporomandibular joint pain. It then transitioned over into other fields including orthopedics and musculoskeletal medicine with the primary goal of promoting a healing response. Platelets are endogenous cells in the blood that respond to injury and trauma by becoming activated and helping with clotting. They also promote an inflammatory response (there is that word again) and release growth factors to start the rebuilding process thus promoting anatomical and functional restoration. The procedure is broken down into two parts. The first involves drawing anywhere from 30-120 cc's of blood and placing it into a centrifuge for multiple spins. The goal is to separate the platelets from the plasma, red blood cells, and white blood cells. The platelets are then injected into the target area or tissue via the use of image guidance including ultrasound or fluoroscopy or a combination of both. These targets may include joints, tendons, ligaments, nerves, skin, and muscle. Immobilization at times is necessary to help with healing and incorporation of the PRP into the tissues. The person then is enrolled into a focused physical therapy and personal training regimen to further enhance recovery.

The following is an example of one of my patients that was helped by this approach. Mr. Shoulder was a 50-year old male with left shoulder pain. He injured himself diving for a softball landing with his left arm outstretched. He presented to clinic after six months of conservative care which failed to improve his symptoms. MRI arthrogram study (imaging after dye placed into the joint) showed evidence of a rotator cuff tear as well as a labral tear. The labrum is the ring of cartilage in the shoulder that provides contact for the joint. The biceps tendon also attaches to this structure. He had been evaluated by an orthopedic surgeon whom recommended surgery, but the patient wanted to exhaust all non-operative treatments prior to moving forward with this recommendation. I evaluated him and we mutually decided to move forward with PRP injection. Approximately 60 cc's of blood was withdrawn which made about 6 cc's of PRP. The substance was injected into the labral tear via fluoroscopy and the rotator cuff tear by ultrasound. The structures around the joint was injected with a prolotherapy solution and platelet poor plasma to help tighten the supporting structures. The patient was placed into a sling for 48 hours and started in an exercise routine soon afterwards. The patient responded well and improved by about 60% initially. We decided to repeat the procedure after 6 months due to ongoing symptoms. The patient improved about 90-95% at the one-year mark and avoided surgery, time off of work, and a painful rehabilitation program.

This was a step up from prolotherapy with a greater boost for healing with fewer injections necessary. Typical for this injection treatment process to require 1-2 injections to provide response and benefit. Research studies have shown that the response tends to increase the further away that you get from the injection. Meaning that patients three months out from the injection were better than one month out; and patients six months out were better than those whom were three months out. This is a fact that needs to be explained in detail to the patient as an education piece prior to the procedure. This is counter to a typical steroid injection which provides relief within 1-2 weeks but only last 4-6 weeks. This procedure was another step in the proper direction for restoring structure, strength, health, and vitality.

PRP injections are helpful for multiple musculoskeletal and orthopedic diagnoses. It can be used for osteoarthritis with the best response found in the knee. It has utility in tendon injuries such as a rotator cuff tear (shoulder), lateral epicondylitis (tennis elbow), Achilles (lower leg/ankle), and the hamstring (proximal leg/buttock). It has shown efficacy in treating ligament injuries including the medial collateral ligament (inside portion of the knee) and the ulnar collateral ligament of the elbow (inside portion of the elbow common in baseball pitchers). The intervention may also be of benefit for disc abnormalities in the spine (the small donuts of tissue between the vertebral bodies) and the facet joints (connections between bones in the back). The PRP can also become activated releasing the contents of the platelets forming a substance called platelet lysate. This material may then be used as a potent anti-inflammatory to inject arounds spinal or peripheral nerves to help improve pain and function. This may be substituted for steroid which as we have discussed may have negative effects on health and recovery.

The uses for PRP have also expanded as the procedure has been shown to provide benefit in multiple medical arenas. The procedure can be used for aesthetic and dermatological interventions such as the face (Vampire Facial), the breasts (enhancement and lift), and the hair (for hair loss and to encourage growth). It can be employed in the sexual health area for men and women. The men receive a Priapus shot (P-shot) where the PRP is injected into the penile tissue to help with erectile dysfunction, libido, orgasms, and sexual performance. The women receive the orgasm shot (O-Shot) where the PRP is injected into vagina to help with libido, orgasm, incontinence, painful intercourse, and vaginal atrophy. The treatment may also be used in the infectious disease field to help with superficial infections as it can be antibacterial and thus limiting the side effects of exposure to antibiotics. This intervention may also be used to enhance wound healing and improve the appearance and pain of scars. The mechanism is similar in that it restores the tissue via the release of growth factors, and it improves blood flow which ultimately enhances recovery as well as function. These interventions will all be offered at my practice focusing on functional restoration and rejuvenation.

CHAPTER 6: REGENERATIVE MEDICINE PART III - STEM CELLS

The next facet of the treatment paradigm for regenerative medicine was the introduction of stem cells. Stem cells are biological cells found in multicellular organisms (like humans and other mammals) which can differentiate into other types of cells and/or may divide into more of the same type of cells. Adult stem cells are found in various tissues in the body, and they act as a repair system for the body with the goal of replenishing tissues. For example, stem cells lie in the bone marrow near the end of the bones toward the joint. Microtrauma may occur which stimulates the activation of stem cells which ultimately repair and rejuvenate the joint and thus limiting damage and degeneration. When a mismatch occurs between breakdown and repair, then the patient becomes prone to joint damage including osteoarthritis, bone infarcts (bone death), instability, asymmetry, pain, and dysfunction. Stem cells are present in multiple areas of the body, but the three most common are bone marrow, adipose tissue (fat cells), and blood.

The most common site for the harvesting of adult stem cells would be bone marrow. This procedure involves using a large bore needle to drill down in the bone primarily in the iliac crest or femur and withdrawing about 10 cc's of marrow at six different sites for a total of 60 cc's of solution. The marrow is then centrifuged to obtain the stem cells. They are then injected into the target tissue similar to the way that PRP is done. The utility and indications for stem cells is similar to those treatments in the PRP and Prolotherapy sections which include joints, ligaments, tendons, muscles, nerve, skin, sexual organs, breasts, hair, and discs. There are also processes where the eyes, lungs heart, liver, spinal, cord, and brain may be treated with these cells. Stem cells are also commonly used in treatment of certain cancers including leukemia and multiple myeloma. Prior to treatment, blood work is typically completed including a complete blood count with differential, calcium, phosphorus, alkaline phosphatase, magnesium, N-terminal telopeptide (NTX), vitamin K, and vitamin D levels. These laboratory studies evaluate for diseases of bone including leukemia, multiple myeloma, Paget's disease, and osteoporosis. If there is evidence of cancer, deficiency, or osteopenia/osteoporosis, then the patient may be best treated by amniotic cells. This treatment will be further discussed below.

Stem cells are desirable as a treatment option as they may have a very potent effect in stimulating the healing response for the targeted tissue. Typical need is for 1-2 procedures that may be separated by months to years. Due to the time involved in the harvesting and injection (typically a 2-6 hours), these interventions are the most expensive of the regenerative procedures. There are protocols where prolotherapy injections and PRP injections are done on different days prior to the stem cell procedure to prime the joint for treatment. There are other protocols where prolotherapy and PRP are performed on the same day as the stem cells to augment the procedure. Stem cells tend to diminish as we age and they tend to do so more consistently in women than in men. Certain actions by the patient have the ability to improve the density of stem cells: fasting or intermittent fasting; ingestion of blueberries, green tea, pomegranates, goji berries, and spirulina; and bouts of acute exercise.

Stem cells are advantageous due to multiple reparative mechanisms. They change the environment of the joint from catabolic (breaking down tissue) to anabolic (building tissue). They encourage the release of growth factors and cytokines that result in the recruitment of other cells (paracrine effect) that help with tissue repair and restoration. Stem cells also support tissue remodeling over scar formation. The cells also secrete chemicals that alter the immune response and limit destruction of the joint by macrophages. This also serves to inhibit apoptosis or cell death. This allows the cells to survive longer and exert their positive effects on the target area. The beauty of stem cells in the musculoskeletal realm is that they may differentiate into bone, cartilage, tendon, and ligament tissue.

For those patients that would not be considered candidates for bone marrow harvest due to cancer or osteoporosis, then alternative cells from amniotic fluid or umbilical cord membrane may be used. These substances may be injected into body areas and tissues similar to prolotherapy, PRP, and stem cells. They provide growth factors and other materials to help improve healing. Contrary to their purported claims, these products contain no stem cells and when studied showed only dead cells. Much of this evaluation and laboratory investigation was performed by Dr. Chris Centeno whom has pioneered much of the work and study on regenerative medicine techniques. These products are oftentimes pushed by chiropractors, naturopaths, and acupuncturists as stem cell-based procedures. These claims are misleading and fraudulent due to the aforementioned research. Oftentimes, these interventions are performed without imaging guidance which further limits the efficacy and benefit from the procedure. While these procedures may be helpful in the right circumstance and for the proper patient, consumers need to understand that all treatments are not the same. You also need to understand the training and competency of the physician in providing the most beneficial and cost-effective intervention. The take home message for patients is to do your homework and fully vet your provider and clinic. Ask appropriate questions and if you have concerns, then consider a second opinion.

CHAPTER 7: BUILDING BLOCKS - HORMONES AND SUPPLEMENTS

"Our hormones keep us healthy and when restored to optimal ranges, they keep us energetic and youthful"

—-Dr. Neal Rouzier

I now had new and exciting set of interventional procedures as part of my toolbox to help restore, heal, and regenerate. I still however felt that there were elements missing from fully optimizing patient health, vitality, and recovery. The next part of my personal and professional transformation story materialized at another conference hosted by the AAOM. There was an introductory talk given by Dr. Neal Rouzier about preventative medicine, healthy aging, and hormone replacement. Dr. Rouzier was incredibly engaging and employed a sarcastic humor that drove home his many excellent points in relation to the misinformation in the literature and press about hormone replacement. The discussion opened my eyes to another treatment paradigm and challenged much of the information that we were taught in medical school, residency, and other medical courses. My interest was piqued and I was galvanized to learn more about this life changing plan for altering chronic disease and providing building blocks for healing. I quickly enrolled in the four-part hormone series that Dr. Rouzier runs through Worldlink Medical. The beauty of this learning opportunity was the fact that all of the information presented was evidence-based and validated by the medical literature. The conclusions were compelling and totally focused on patient benefit/outcomes which are buzzwords that many of the insurers are looking at including Medicare. The problem however lies in the fact that these services are typically not covered by insurers and oftentimes they question the medications used and the length of treatment. The issues are not related to efficacy/benefit. They are the result of cost and the negative influence of the pharmaceutical industry. The problem is that natural substances like bio-identical hormones cannot be patented and therefore there is little in the way of profit for using these medications. These companies thus take these molecules and attempt to modify them for financial gain. These drugs oftentimes provide poorer results and may increase potential side effects which at times may be deadly. Examples are the synthetic forms of hormone replacement for women: Premarin (estrogen) and Provera (progestin). These unnatural substances were actually the forms that caused an increase in breast cancer and blood clots and provided the negative press and fear of hormone replacement. The bio-identical forms including estradiol and progesterone have none of these effects, but they are vilified without justification from the literature. For that reason, you as the patient need to be inquisitive and open-minded in an attempt to truly understand the results. All hormones are not the same, and all practitioners are not educated on the capabilities and long-term health benefits of hormone replacement.

In my years of practicing orthopedic medicine, I have seen a number of patients whom had issues with their health. Obesity was a major problem that was negatively affecting a great majority. This disease was placing a great deal of stress on their joints and soft tissues. They had tried a number of diets which were short term fixes but failed to impact the issue long term. They had metabolic syndrome which included hypertension, elevated blood sugars, high triglycerides, low HDL (the good cholesterol), and abdominal obesity. Many were fatigued and lethargic with poor sleep habits. Stress levels were elevated and from a mental health standpoint they were depressed and anxious with little in the way of drive. Libido was low and they were having sexual dysfunction issues. They were having concerns about memory loss and clarity of thought (brain fog). They were having difficulties with their personal relationships including their significant other and friends which further isolated them placing them in harm's way. They were also on a number of pharmaceutical medications treating their symptoms but failing to change their overall health. These medications also had side effects which were further negatively impacting their vitality and life enjoyment. I had little in the way of help for all of these medical problems, and they were all having an impact on their improvement and recovery from their orthopedic obstacles. Hormone and supplement optimization allowed me to address many of these predicaments and allowed me to provide a solution for most. It also helped to provide the foundation and building blocks to accentuate and augment the response to regenerative medicine procedures.

Hormones are chemical substances produced by endocrine glands such as the thyroid, pituitary, pineal, ovaries, testicles, and adrenals. These chemicals regulate all essential functions of the human body including temperature, growth, reproduction, recovery, healing, immunity, and aging. When hormones are optimal and balanced, the body functions well from a physical, psychological, and emotional standpoint. When hormones are altered due to injury, disease, age, or medications; then patients exhibit a noticeable decline and deterioration. At that stage, we are existing instead of living. We are surviving instead of thriving. Providing preventative medicine and replacing deficiency with bio-identical hormones alters this path and allows us to restore the patient to ideal health and function. In the upcoming paragraphs, I will provide a brief synopsis of each of the major hormones that are typically evaluated and optimized. These will include testosterone, estrogen, progesterone, thyroid, DHEA, vitamin D, and growth hormone.

CHAPTER 8: TESTOSTERONE-ESSENTIAL FOR BOTH MEN AND WOMEN

Testosterone is a hormone that is essential for ideal function in both men and women. In men, the hormone is produced in the testes (95%) and the adrenals (5%). In women, it is primarily produced in the ovaries and adrenals.

In men, lower testosterone levels cause hypogonadism or andropause. The hallmarks of this disease process include fatigue, depression, erectile dysfunction, decreased libido, sarcopenia (muscle atrophy), functional weakness, and a loss of confidence/drive. These patients also have an increased risk of heart disease, osteoporosis, cholesterol elevation, mental decline, and Alzheimer's dementia. Optimizing levels of testosterone typically treat this combination of issues and protect against chronic diseases and health problems that increase health costs and increase the risk for disability. It also limits the need for treatment of high blood pressure, cholesterol disease, erectile dysfunction, osteoporosis, depression, and dementia. This also serves to limit polypharmacy, reduce costs, minimize side effects and cross reactivity of these drugs, and improve function. Think about it, one hormone with multiple benefits limits the need for multiple expensive drugs with questionable efficacy and potential negative side effects. This is a trade I am definitely willing to take and so should YOU! The hormone may be taken in three different forms. The first is a daily or weekly injection of testosterone which is typically self-administered after education from myself or one of our other practitioners. The second is a topical cream that is placed on the scrotum twice a day which maximizes absorption. The third is a pellet that inserted into the skin and soft tissues above the buttock on either side. All of these approaches are well tolerated and ideal for reaching optimal levels. Blood work is typically done after the initial consultation to obtain baseline levels. Once treatment begins, then levels are commonly checked every six weeks until optimal levels have been reached and/or symptoms have resolved. At that point, levels are then done every six months to confirm ideal levels and/or to adjust dosages. This pattern is similar for the other hormones that are replaced and will be discussed in the coming chapters.

In women, testosterone is vital for a number of functions and it is equally as important for them as it is for men. Testosterone is described as the "feel good" hormone as it improves mood, energy, libido, and an overall sense of well-being. Testosterone is important for sexual function including clitoral sensitivity, lubrication, energy, and desire. It is helpful as an aesthetic agent as it prevents wrinkles and skin thinning from collagen loss. It also benefits musculoskeletal health limiting muscle loss and atrophy, maintaining strength and function with a concomitant exercise routine, and preventing osteoporosis and potential vertebral, hip, and wrist fractures (along with estrogen/DHEA/growth hormone). The testosterone and estrogen combination also has been shown to have beneficial effects on the cardiovascular system including vasodilation and improvement in HDL levels (good cholesterol) and triglyceride levels (decreases visceral fat). Testosterone replacement is also vital in treating the hot flashes and night sweats associated with perimenopause (pre-menopause) and menopause. Testosterone treatments are also helpful in women that have been treated for breast cancer as they are apoptotic (kill cancer cells) and diminish the stimulation of breast tissue. Progesterone has a very similar effect and should be given concurrently with testosterone in these patients. Testosterone may be provided to women in four different forms. The first is injection on either a daily or weekly basis. The second is a cream placed on the vagina/labia on a daily basis which may also help with lubrication, vaginal atrophy, urinary incontinence, and clitoral sensitivity. The third is a pellet that is inserted in the soft tissues of the buttock. The fourth is a micronized capsule formulated by a compounding pharmacy. Laboratory studies are performed the same as those outlined in the above paragraph.

CHAPTER 9: THYROID HORMONE-MORE THAN ENERGY AND METABOLISM

Thyroid hormone deficiencies are fairly common and consistently undertreated in our current healthcare system. The disconnect occurs as physicians fail to treat symptoms of hypothyroidism and only focus on the numbers. The numbers used however are insufficient for providing a diagnosis and treatment plan. The medications used are also inadequate to optimally treat the problem and provide relief of the symptoms for a thyroid gland functioning sub-optimally. The thyroid is a small butterfly shaped gland in the front of the neck above the trachea. The thyroid gland is stimulated to produce active hormone (T3 or triiodothyronine) and inactive hormone (T4 or thyroxine) by a chemical produced in the anterior pituitary gland called TSH (thyrotropin). Thyroid hormone is integral for multiple life processes including metabolism, temperature regulation, and cerebral function. Hypothyroid or deficiency symptoms may include fatigue, memory impairment, weight gain, depression, temperature imbalance, dry skin, brittle nails, constipation, and menstrual irregularities (in women). These issues are primarily seen as a part of the natural aging process by the mainstream healthcare community. For that reason, hypothyroidism is consistently undertreated. The problems also typically overlap with other issues such as andropause, menopause, sleep deprivation, depression, anxiety, and cognitive decline which further complicates the treatment.

Thyroid deficiency affects 10% of men and 20% of women although these numbers in my opinion are low. There are many more that have symptoms and subclinical hypothyroidism that fail to receive treatment. These issues are often missed due to the fact that typical evaluation by medical professionals primarily involves evaluation of TSH and at times free T4. TSH is a poor measure of thyroid function as the normal range is so vast. The TSH and free T4 also fail to assess the active form of the hormone which is free T3. Normal free T4 levels also may be misleading as this needs to be converted to free T3 for activity via the enzyme deiodinase. If this enzyme is low or functioning abnormally, then no conversion occurs and the symptoms rear their ugly head. This is the reason that the commercially available medications including Synthroid and Levoxyl fail to improve symptoms in upwards of 15-20% of patients. They contain only T4 and must be converted to the active form in the body. This is the main reason to use a combination drug like Armour or Nature-Throid which contain both T3 and T4. The pharmaceutical industry in their infinite wisdom has attempted to discredit these products in hopes of sustaining profits. Similar to our current presidential administration, they use fear, lies, and denials (of the evidence-based science) to carry out this injustice. This practice is pervasive in medicine and society as a whole and it needs to stop. Facts and truth matter, and they need to trump (pun intended) profit and power as motivation for actions.

I will provide an example to illustrate many of these points. I had a patient by the name of Ima Tired. The patient was a 52 year-old female whom presented with a hip issue. As we discussed her issue, it became clear that her primary problems included weight gain, fatigue, depression, brittle nails, and hair loss. She had discussed these issues with her primary MD whom ran a TSH study as well as iron studies and a CBC (complete blood count). All of these studies were normal. She was treated with an antidepressant and advised to lose weight without a particular plan do so.

She was also told that tiredness was a part of ageing and life. We discussed these issues in detail and I advised her that it was likely her thyroid. I ran a complete thyroid panel and indeed her TSH was normal, but her free T3 was very low. I started her on Armour Thyroid and eventually adjusted the dosage to the point where her above symptoms resolved and thus her levels were optimized. The patient was much happier and was able to lose 20 lbs. in six months with hormone treatment, nutrition advice and exercise. Her hip issues resolved with a course of physical therapy and a strengthening program. The only person that was unhappy was her primary MD. She called demanding that the Armour Thyroid should be discontinued due to the potential side effects of its use. She also was upset as she did not feel that the patient had thyroid issues due to the results of her limited work-up. I discussed my work-up which included an extensive history (symptoms), physical exam (clinical), and laboratory study. I also discussed her positive results in relation to weight loss, improvements in energy and mood, and resolution of her nail and hair issues. Her hip issues had also resolved with conservative treatment, and she had discontinued her antidepressant. I also sent her multiple articles on thyroid and the many benefits of replacing this hormone. She really didn't care as was she totally focused on the potential issues with Armour and the diagnosis (incorrect per her evaluation). She also made a statement which typified modern medicine and confirmed that I was on to something and doing the right thing. She noted that all her patients were tired and that this was just part of getting older and ageing. I told her to please send those folks over to see me, and I would happily treat them and improve their quality of life and health. Not surprisingly, she hung up on me. I therefore tell patients (you) that I am treating you and not any of their doctors. If their doctors do not understand the treatment

and the literature, then I will be unable to change their mind.
I educate you that many of my treatments will be unpopular
with the healthcare community as a whole, but that the
reason that you are in my office asking for help is that these
mainstream treatments have failed. Therefore, you as the
patient need to be inquisitive and a critical thinker focusing
on your specific health issues and needs. In turn, I will
definitely return the favor and guide you towards the
treatment(s) that will provide the most benefit.

CHAPTER 10: ESTROGEN-THE ONE THAT STARTED IT ALL

Estrogen restoration is the treatment that initiated the field of hormone replacement therapy. This hormone is responsible for a number of health benefits in women, but also in men. The loss of this hormone during menopause in women and with age in men has many negative and deleterious effects. These include an increased risk of heart disease, stroke, cholesterol abnormalities, Alzheimer's disease, memory loss, osteoporosis, skin atrophy, depression, weight gain, vaginal atrophy (women), and urinary tract atrophy (women). These problems thus cause a significant burden on the healthcare system and increase costs astronomically due to polypharmacy (multiple drugs), ER visits and hospitalizations, surgeries (cardiac and orthopedic as examples), procedures (cardiac catheterizations and kyphoplasties), nursing home stays, and lost work days for caregivers. These are issues that may be easily avoided today and in the future with appropriate treatment including estrogen replacement (and progesterone for women).

Estrogen has been unjustly vilified in the medical community and by the press. The panic started after the Women's Health Initiative (WHI) study. This study was completed using the synthetic forms of estrogen (Premarin) and progestins (Provera) and not the bio-identical equivalents of estradiol and progesterone. The study actually showed that the initiation of Premarin at menopause showed a reduced risk of heart disease and stroke. There was also no increased risk of breast cancer with Premarin alone. There was an increased risk of blood clots with Premarin. The bad actor in the study was the Provera. This synthetic progestin increased the risk of breast cancer and therefore was the culprit for the rise in this disease (not the Premarin). The Provera also further increased the risk of blood clots, pulmonary embolus (blood clot in the lungs), heart attack, and stroke. Subsequent studies have shown no increased risk for breast cancer, blood clot, stroke, or heart attack for the bio-identical hormones estradiol and progesterone. In fact, these hormones have been shown to be protective if started at menopause. Despite the data supporting the positive effects of bio-identical hormones and the negative and potentially dangerous effects of synthetic hormones, they (synthetic hormones) remain on the market. The pharmaceutical industry has again duped the public, and the medical community as a whole has bought into the lie without protest. Profits again are placed at a higher priority than the health of the population at large. The evidence-based scientific information is again ignored and harmful effects follow. This vicious cycle further fuels the drug industry to provide drugs to treat symptoms instead of providing cures. As noted in the aforementioned chapters, this seems to be a common theme and refrain for the status quo and a continuation of the medical industrial complex. It is thus our job (me as the physician and you as the patient) to break this cycle and trumpet facts over distortions and deceitful marketing.

Estrogen in men is incredibly important as it protects against many of the negative effects that also afflict women. These include cardiovascular disease, stroke, cholesterol abnormalities, osteoporosis, dementia, Alzheimer's disease, increased visceral fat/weight gain, and skin thinning. Estrogen in men is produced by the aromatization (conversion) of testosterone to estrogen. These adverse effects may become particularly pronounced when either testosterone is diminished or estrogen conversion is blocked.

The former may occur with age and the subsequent decrease in testosterone levels or with chemical castration via Lupron (decreases testosterone and estrogen production) and Casodex (block testosterone receptors) to treat prostate cancer. The treatment of testosterone loss due to age would be testosterone replacement. The treatment for prostate cancer would be to start oral estrogen as it provides two benefits. These would include improving symptoms of estrogen loss and treating the prostate cancer. The latter (estrogen blockade) is advocated by the bodybuilding community and some wellness organizations as a way to maximize the activity of testosterone. This action is commonly executed by the prescription medicine Arimidex which is an aromatase inhibitor that blocks the conversion of testosterone to estrogen. Intuitively, it seems to make sense that optimal testosterone is good, then having more must be better. It also seems ideal to limit the production of the female hormone estrogen when the male hormone effects are trying to be maximized. Studies however have shown that blocking estrogen is a terrible idea and significantly increases side effects. These include heart attack, stroke, cholesterol abnormalities, vascular disease (narrowing of the arteries and veins), increased visceral fat, diabetes, hypertension, gynecomastia (man boobs), and low libido. These effects seem counterintuitive but they have been borne out in multiple studies. If you look at estrogen levels in men in their teenage years and in their twenties, they run in the 100-200 range as testosterone levels are optimal from endogenous production. At no time do we block estrogen in these age groups; yet, we would want to negatively affect it in these older populations when we attempt to maximize testosterone. It makes no sense and thus we need to follow the science and not "bro science" (that purported in gyms and in online chat rooms to be true). All of these interventions (adding estrogen or testosterone) or lack thereof (not blocking estrogen) have been demonstrated to improve the overall well-being and longevity of the patient (you).

CHAPTER 11:
PROGESTERONE-THE YANG TO THE YIN OF ESTROGEN

Progesterone is a hormone that is the natural partner to estrogen in women. Progesterone in menstruating females typically rises in the second half (last fourteen days) of the cycle to prepare the lining of the uterus for a potential fertilized egg. If no fertilization occurs, then progesterone drops and bleeding occurs. If pregnancy occurs, then the progesterone levels remain elevated to carry the child to term. If progesterone levels drop, then this causes difficulty carrying a baby to full term and may lead to miscarriage. These issues may be particularly pronounced in women with polycystic ovarian syndrome whom consistently have low or absent progesterone levels. Replacing this hormone along with a number of interventions too numerous to list here may allow these women to carry a child to term thus limiting the need for expensive fertility drugs and specialty obstetrics and gynecology clinics.

Ideal levels of progesterone provide the yang to estrogen's yin. Progesterone optimization offers multiple health benefits to women. These include improvements in cardiovascular parameters, bone health, lipids, mood, quality of life, and contentment. Maximizing this hormone also provides protection against breast cancer, uterine cancer, fibrocystic breast disease, and vaginal atrophy. This hormone is also the first line treatment for premenstrual syndrome (PMS) and menstrual migraines. High dose treatment is also helpful in managing endometrial hyperplasia (thickening of the cells in the lining of the uterus) which may cause abnormal bleeding and become a precursor for cancer. Bio-identical progesterone has no known side effects. This fact is in direct contrast to the synthetic progestin Provera. Provera causes significant side effects including breast cancer, weight gain, water retention and bloating, breast tenderness, blood clots, heart attack, stroke, and depression. The only thing that it protects against is uterine cancer. Therefore, progesterone and Provera are not the same molecule and lumping them together must stop. The science is clear and bio-identical progesterone has a distinct advantage and should be the drug of choice for women requiring hormone replacement. The fact that Provera is still on the market with the multitude of side effects and deaths caused by this drug is reprehensible. Women are constantly placed in harm's way with the combination of Premarin and Provera when safer and more effective alternatives are readily available. This is the pharmaceutical industry and the complicit doctors at their worst. Profits and propaganda over the health and welfare of women. If any healthcare practitioner attempts to prescribe Premarin and Provera to you, turn and run to our office. I will treat you according to the literature in an attempt to optimize your health and vitality and formulate **A NEW YOU!**

These points are best illustrated by the following patient that I treated whom was despondent when she presented to my office. I will call her Mrs. Menopause. She was a 57-year old female who initially complained of low back pain. Diving deeper, the patient noted issues with memory and concentration, sleep, vaginal dryness, low libido, hot flashes and night sweats, and skin changes. Her energy levels were low and she was depressed/emotionally labile. She had a recent DEXA (bone density) scan which showed her to be osteopenic with a loss of bone density. She was started on an antidepressant by her primary MD which caused side effects including nausea, constipation, and anxiety. She was also started on the benzodiazepine Ativan to help with sleep and anxiety. This medication made her feel dizzy and drunk. No lab work was done to assess her medical or hormone status. No medications were started or exercises prescribed to combat the osteopenia/bone loss. The back pain was mild and no specific treatment had been started for this disorder. She was "a basket case" and needed help pronto. I ordered a battery of blood work to assess her medical status, hormone levels, and bone health. I also ordered a urinalysis to assess for infection and/or renal disease. X-rays were also obtained of her lumbar spine and pelvis. The studies showed no sign of infection or anemia. The NTX level was elevated consistent with bone loss. Her estrogen, progesterone, testosterone, thyroid, and Vitamin D levels were all low and suboptimal. Her FSH (follicle stimulating hormone) and LH (luteinizing hormone) levels were such (along with her low estrogen and progesterone levels) that she had reached menopause. She was started on oral estradiol, progesterone, thyroid (Armour), DHEA, and Vitamin D. She was also started on a testosterone cream placed on the vagina at night. The patient significantly improved and her symptoms resolved such that she stopped her antidepressant and Ativan. She was started in a physical therapy and chiropractic regimen for her back issues. Repeat DEXA scan and NTX levels showed her bone density had returned to normal. These results are common and typical for the woman that has reached menopause with symptoms. This treatment has also improved her long-term health and survival.

CHAPTER 12: DHEA-THE MARKER OF LONGEVITY AND LIFESPAN

DHEA (dehydroepiandrosterone) is a hormone unto itself as well as a hormone precursor that has the ability to convert into estrogen, progesterone, and testosterone. DHEA is formed in the adrenal gland and has the effect of shifting catabolic (breakdown) processes to anabolic (building) activities. DHEA is the most abundant hormone in the body with multiple health benefits. The most interesting fact associated with this hormone and the primary reason for monitoring levels lies in the fact that it is the best biochemical marker of age. A New England Journal of Medicine article from 1986 concluded that DHEA levels were inversely related to death from any cause and death from cardiovascular disease in men over 50. Thus, higher levels of DHEA are associated with increased longevity whereas lower levels are predictive of early mortality. Therefore, overall morbidity and mortality is directly related to DHEA levels. To again quote Dr Rouzier, "What do you want your levels to be?" The answer would be optimal.

DHEA has multiple positive effects on the body for overall health, healthy aging and longevity. It serves to increase lipolysis (fat breakdown) thus reducing visceral fat. This effect is common with many of the hormones as we have seen in previous discussions, and one of the major reasons that chronic disease is significantly reduced with hormone optimization (see above and below). DHEA has a profound effect on immune function thus reducing the risk of acute and chronic illness. For this reason, the risk of cancer is also reduced with optimal levels of DHEA. It works as an anti-inflammatory and therefore has indications for treating autoimmune disorders such as lupus and rheumatoid arthritis. It also has benefits for patients suffering from osteoarthritis. It reduces IL-6 which is a pro-inflammatory cytokine which has many deleterious effects on the body. This list of conditions where IL-6 is elevated includes diabetes, atherosclerosis, multiple myeloma, prostate cancer, and Behcet's disease, and DHEA thus is beneficial for these conditions via this dampening effect. It improves mood, energy levels, and memory and helps to guard against Alzheimer's dementia. DHEA improves bone health and is part of the comprehensive treatment plan for patients with osteopenia/osteoporosis (including estrogen, progesterone, testosterone, growth hormone, vitamin D, Vitamin K, magnesium, and strength training). DHEA also has the effect of controlling cortisol levels thus reducing the stress and other negative effects hypothalamic-pituitary-adrenal axis (HPA axis) disorders.

DHEA is typically taken twice a day in both men and women. Side effects include acne and hirsutism (hairiness). Both of these effects may be reduced and/or resolved via dose reduction. Levels are assessed via bloodwork and typically adjusted up or down after six weeks of initiating therapy. After optimal levels are obtained, DHEA will then typically be checked at six-month intervals. In summary, DHEA treatment helps reduce the risk of cancer, cardiovascular disease, Alzheimer's dementia, osteoporosis, autoimmune disorders, osteoarthritis, and HPA axis disorders.

CHAPTER 13: GROWTH HORMONE-THE CONTROVERSIAL AND MISUNDERSTOOD HORMONE

Growth hormone (GH) is an endogenous substance that is synthesized, stored, and secreted by the pituitary gland. Like most hormones, growth hormone has multiple varied functions in the body. It is typically secreted at night to stimulate growth, repair, and cell regeneration. It also has a profound effect on bone health as it stimulates osteoblasts and bone growth via retention of calcium. It is in fact the most potent substance that may be used to fight bone loss. It is also released in stressful or fight or flight reactions and raises the levels of glucose, free fatty acids, and IGF-1.

Deficiency of growth hormone has been shown to overlap with aging. The reasons are many and varied but primarily focus on the loss of vital function. These include bone health issues, reduced exercise tolerance, and sarcopenia (loss of muscle mass). These conditions increase the risk for fall, fracture, impairment, and disability. Loss of GH also increases fat deposition and insulin resistance. Dyslipidemia occurs which raises LDL which may be problematic in patients with prior heart attacks and strokes. Overall, there is an increased morbidity and mortality from all cardiovascular causes with diminishing levels. Cognitive decline and the risk of Alzheimer's disease increases with decreasing GH levels. All of these deleterious effects have a negative impact on quality of life.

Growth hormone has many beneficial effects and therefore may be of benefit improving health span and longevity. It maximizes bone health and reduces the risk of osteopenia/osteoporosis. It increases muscle mass via hypertrophy of existing cells and potentially via creating new ones. It increases protein synthesis which helps with repair and recovery from exercise and/or injury. It plays a role in homeostasis thus maintaining an equilibrium in our bodies limiting entropy and chaos. It stimulates the immune system and helps to fight acute and chronic inflammation. It helps with the conversion of T4 (inactive precursor) to T3 (active thyroid hormone). It increases lipolysis and thus reduces visceral fat and its negative health consequences such as diabetes mellitus and metabolic syndrome. It also serves to maintain the size of all organs including the heart. This has the benefit of maintaining and increasing cardiac output thus reducing the risk and negative effects of congestive heart failure.

Growth hormone levels are measured indirectly by looking at IGF-1 levels in the blood. IGF-1 (insulin like growth factor 1) is produced via the effect of GH on the liver. IGF-1 has growth-stimulating effects on multiple tissues in the body as outlined in the above discussion. Growth hormone is typically administered via daily injection. Levels are typically checked every six weeks until optimization has occurred. GH may typically take upwards of six months to start showing benefit. Side effects to the medication may include edema, arthralgias, myalgias, and carpal tunnel syndrome. These effects are primarily due to the antinatriuretic effect of GH on the kidney and thus fluid is retained. The main drawback of using growth hormone ion a long-term basis is the cost of the medication. For this reason, alternatives including sermorelin (growth hormone releasing hormone-GHRH analog) may be used which provide similar results and are more cost-effective for the patient.

Growth hormone (and to a lesser degree testosterone) have become common negative targets in the media due to their use by celebrities and patients for their anti-aging effects; and sports-talk radio due to abuse and potential performance enhancement in athletes. While these substances are banned for use by all professional, college, and Olympic athletes, the information put forth in discussion of these substances is oftentimes erroneous and just plain wrong. This only serves to further cloud the picture and pollute the message for potential use of these hormones by the patient whom is looking for the health benefits. In the right setting and with proper prescription via a trained physician or health professional, these hormones have a place in the treatment of multiple health issues. I would also bet that in our lifetimes that the professional sports leagues will come around to the idea of physician assisted hormone replacement for their constituents. Treatment will likely have the effect of limiting injury and the number of lost games due to health problems. Bio-identical hormone replacement would also likely have the effect of extending the careers of many of the stars of sport further maintaining interest in the game by the fan. Money talks, and, ultimately, I think that these restrictions will be relaxed and a scientific program of treatment and replacement will be a mainstay of every team. This will significantly reduce cheating due to the constant monitoring of levels and drug amounts, thus creating a level playing field for all players involved and reducing any laboratory advantage. I also believe that this will happen for cannabis (marijuana) as the medical benefits for this "sacred plant" far outweigh the negatives. This however will be a discussion for another book.

CHAPTER 14: VITAMIN D-THE SUPPLEMENT THAT IS A HORMONE

Vitamin D is an excellent supplement but also works in the body primarily as a hormone. It is a steroid hormone that is generated in the skin via sun exposure from cholesterol. Vitamin D may also be supplied by food and by supplementation. Vitamin D has multiple positive effects on the body similar to the other hormones that we have discussed. Vitamin D plays a significant role in bone health by increasing the intestinal absorption of calcium, magnesium, and phosphate. It also promotes the healthy growth and remodeling of bone as optimal levels Vitamin D are paramount to the proactive and reactive treatments for these disorders. It also allows for proper functioning of parathyroid hormone which helps to maintain ideal levels of calcium in the blood. Vitamin D works to maintain muscle size, strength, and function via minimizing sarcopenia and muscle atrophy. This also has the benefit of reducing falls and the resulting trauma and disability that may occur. It is also helpful in improving overactive bladder, pulmonary function, macular degeneration, and cognitive decline. It has also been shown to decrease the risk of breast, colorectal, ovarian, renal, pancreatic, and prostate cancer. High/optimal levels of vitamin D have been associated with a substantial decrease in cardiovascular disease, diabetes mellitus (type II), and metabolic syndrome. Vitamin D treatment also provides benefit for depression and reduces all-cause mortality by 7%. Optimal levels have also been shown to combat and treat the deleterious effects of autoimmune diseases such as rheumatoid arthritis, SLE, Crohn's disease, ulcerative colitis, leaky gut, Hashimoto's thyroiditis, diabetes mellitus, eczema, and Alzheimer's dementia (described as diabetes mellitus Type III).

Vitamin D comes in two supplemental forms. The first is ergocalciferol or Vitamin D2 which is metabolized to 25-hydroxyergocalciferol. The second is cholecalciferol which is Vitamin D3. This form is metabolized in the liver to calcifediol (25-hydroxycholecalciferol). These two metabolites call 25-hydroxyvitamin D or 25(OH)D. These levels are measures via blood work to determine the Vitamin D level. Calcifediol is further hydroxylated in the kidneys to form calcitriol (1,25-dihydroxycholecalciferol) which is the biologically active form of Vitamin D. Typical doses for optimization are 5,000 to 10,000 international units per day. The body may formulate Vitamin D from 7-dehydrocholesterol from reaction via UVB radiation via the sun. Exposure to the sun for 5-10 minutes upwards of 2-3 times per week (without sunscreen) typically is sufficient for optimal Vitamin D levels. Food sources of Vitamin D include cod liver oil, herring, swordfish, mushrooms, sardines, tuna, fortified milk, and eggs. Ideal levels range from 60-100 nmol/L. Levels above 100 may become necessary for patients with severe deficiency and rarely cause side effects.

Symptoms of Vitamin D deficiency include frequent illness and/or infection due to immune system suppression, fatigue, bone pain, mental health issues, impaired wound healing, hair loss, and myofascial pain. These are common problems that afflict patients that I assess on a daily basis. Chronic deficiency of Vitamin D may result in obesity, diabetes, hypertension, depression fibromyalgia, chronic fatigue syndrome, osteoporosis, and neurodegenerative disorders. For example, patients with diffuse muscle pain/fibromyalgia respond well to Vitamin D optimization (as well as thyroid, growth hormone, and testosterone maximization). Impaired wound healing and hair loss may also be treated by PRP injections (discussed previously) along with Vitamin D. These examples thus illustrate the theme expressed throughout the pages in this book that treatment plans are multifactorial and typically require time to fully manage the problem. This conforms with my overall philosophy that everything matters and is intertwined in the fabric of disease and dysfunction. Therefore, knowledge is power for both myself and the patient and my education has ultimately provided a plethora of tools and options for management.

CHAPTER 15: THE VILLAIN/VILLAINS OF OUR HEALTHCARE DRAMA

The best movies, books, television programs, and sporting events are enjoyable and compelling as there is typically an adversary to despise. This enemy sets up conflict and such that there is a negative force or hurdle that needs to be overcome or slayed. This current saga is no different and if I stopped with this chapter, then it would be considered a tragedy. The villain/villains of this epic story are the current pillars of the healthcare industry: the health insurance carriers, the pharmaceutical industry, large hospital systems, healthcare conglomerates, the food industry, the government, and the majority of healthcare providers. This seems like a long and profound list of problem children. It also contains a number of members whom would typically be viewed as friends and not foes. The truth however is that the key members of the industrial healthcare complex are the key contributors to chronic disease and poor overall health. The main goal of these players is not wellness, prevention, evidence-based science, function, restoration, fitness, vitality, nutrition, or longevity. These things limit disease and promote health and well-being. It seems as though these goals would be the thrust of treatment and the ideal outcome for individual and group healthcare interventions. In a Utopian society, this would be true. In our capitalistic world, special interests take hold and the primary focus becomes profit as opposed to health optimization. In other words, healthy people need less care and services which equals less profit. Sick people need more care and treatments which equals more money and more profits. Therefore, our current system of treatment has been described by many pundits as Sick Care as opposed to healthcare. Thus, there is an infinite number of people whom need office visits, prescription drugs, surgeries, equipment, imaging, procedures, labs, hospital stays, rehabilitation, and nursing home stays. While many of these evaluations or treatments may be helpful or necessary at some point in a person's life, the overall volume has hit critical mass and is overwhelming the system which will ultimately collapse in the future due to bankruptcy and a lack of resources.

This volume is also overwhelming our healthcare providers to the point where 50% of our physicians are burned out. This leads to depression, anger, stress, hopelessness, and disillusionment. Unfortunately, this leads to physician suicide which is on the rise as is suicide as a whole in all age groups in our society. Thus, our physicians are unable to adequately treat their patients due to their own problems and attitudes. I had reached this stage in 2016 and knew that I needed to change and look for a different path which aligned more with my beliefs and my education. These tenets included regenerative orthopedic medicine, fitness and exercise, bio-identical hormone replacement, functional medicine, nutrition, aesthetics, sexual health, psychological well-being, and vitality. These tenets however fly in the face of the plans of the aforementioned villains which serve to quell evidence-based treatments to increase profits. They spew forth misinformation and half-truths which in an Orwellian way (see George Orwell and 1984) attempt to brainwash the masses (patients and physicians) to their way of thinking. The falsehoods are perpetuated and then become dogma when in reality they are primarily only urban legends. These issues will be further highlighted and delineated with specific examples to illustrate my points.

The health insurance industry has become focused on managing cost as opposed to improving health, morbidity (illness), and mortality (death). All of the major companies (Blue Cross/Aetna/United/Cigna) are publicly traded and therefore they are more focused on answering to their shareholders as opposed to their clients (patients). Premiums continue to increase anywhere from 10-20% seemingly on a yearly basis. The deductibles (amount paid by the patient) also have dramatically increased to the point that the patient is otherwise on the hook for all of their health care costs. The only positives to having coverage are the negotiated discounts and catastrophic evasion (from major injury and subsequent bankruptcy). For example, I have a health insurance policy with an unnamed insurance company (United Healthcare) for my family of four (myself, wife, and two kids). We are all in reasonable health and attempt to optimize our wellness and vitality. My premium per month is $1500 while my deductible is $8000 per family and $4000 per individual. In simple terms, I would pay $26,000 this year for healthcare prior to United Healthcare paying a dime. This policy also fails to cover any dental care for my wife or myself. The cost is not the only issue. United still has the right to review and potentially deny care as prescribed or ordered by my doctors which means I have no control over the disbursement of the funds even though this is my money. In my opinion, this is reprehensible and makes it difficult to justify the cost and the hassle. I would rather pay cash and direct my resources to care that I deem appropriate as opposed to another entity collecting my money and determining how it may be directed. This is the reason that cash-based businesses or hybrid businesses (cash and insurance combination) like mine will increase and flourish in the future. Patients are turned off by this current model which negatively impacts their bank accounts, pays for little to no care, restricts choice, and fails to improve health or longevity. This is not sustainable and this alienation of affection will continue to drive patients to search for alternatives, thus I'm writing this book to provide a call to action and a solution (for you).

The pharmaceutical industry is another player in the circus we call healthcare. This is another group that serves the interests of themselves and their shareholders first. If patients improve or get better, then that is an added bonus. Drugs are big business and are focused on profits as opposed to altruistic goals of solving healthcare problems. From Forbes magazine, the total revenue of the global pharmaceutical market in 2015 was $1.05 trillion. Nearly half of the total, $515 billion, was collected from the United States and Canada. These two countries however comprise only 7% of the world's population. Thus, we as Americans pay significantly more for our drugs than the rest of the world. We spend $1443 on drugs per person in the United States which is by far the highest in the world. These drugs treat every symptom known to man including some fabricated syndromes to justify a use for these medications. Yet, we are no healthier than the other countries in the world despite our consumption of drugs and our healthcare. Per the World Health Organization, the United States (US) ranked 37th in the world in regard to quality of health systems. The life expectancy in the US also decreased for the third year in a row which is a concerning trend. The volume of medications on the market has only served to make us sicker secondary to side effects, lack of efficacy, and the cost. For example, statin drugs like Lipitor have been pushed to control cholesterol and limit the negative effects of heart disease and stroke. This group of medications however have not been shown to be useful in the primary prevention of either one of these problems. They also have side effects which include muscle pain, neuropathy, brain fog, and depression. In addition, they also have a negative effect on the formation of sex hormones as this process requires cholesterol as the building block. Statins as a class have also been shown to increase breast cancer risk, and the risk is higher than hormone replacement with estrogen and progesterone (whether it was bioidentical or synthetic). Funny, but we hear nothing from the press, media, or prescribing physicians on this fact when these medications are given out like candy. The industry has also been very successful in limiting the use of cheaper generic medications via contracts with third party payers (ie. the insurance companies discussed above). At times, the copayments for covered drugs are higher than the out of pocket costs for cheaper and equally effective medications. Another example where somebody is spending your money instead of you and negatively affecting your wallet and your health.

Large healthcare conglomerates and large healthcare specialty organizations also play a role in the Psycho Circus (props to the band Kiss and check iTunes for the song). The goal for both is to swallow as many practices, locations, providers, patients, and employees to increase clout and negotiating power. For instance, large hospital systems like Cleveland Clinic, Mayo Clinic, and Carolinas Medical Center (now Atrium Health) perform this gluttonous acquisition strategy to provide leverage against health insurance companies and employers in contract negotiations to maximize market share and profits. They also thus increase the total number of office visits, imaging studies (MRI, CT scans, Ultrasounds, X-rays), surgeries, hospital stays, and facility fees. Large single specialty and multispecialty groups do the same thing to help with negotiations with insurance companies, hospitals, surgery centers, employers, pharmacies, etc. in hopes of attaining the same goal. The main outcomes of these giant companies are typically detrimental for the healthcare system. They serve to increase cost for the consumer due to lack of competition. The feel of the care is very corporate and oftentimes lacks personalization and empathy. In effect, the patient feels like a number (shout out to Creedence Clearwater Revival) and a cash cow for the entity. Not coincidentally, the physicians are treated the same way where they are treated as a cog in the wheel and also a cash cow. This also serves to limit the voice and ingenuity of the physician and physician group(s) due to the sheer size of the entity and the fact that approval needs to come from multiple committees and layers. This negatively affects the mental and physical health of the providers and staff as they have little say in the running of their own practices and the services offered. These issues further erode the quality of care that patients receive, and this leads to dissatisfaction for all of those involved. Smaller groups like mine are more nimble and able to adapt to the changes in the healthcare world. We also understand that you as the patient are the backbone of the practice, and for that reason you will be treated as a unique individual with your own unique problems. You choose what you want your healthcare to be and how it is delivered. My advice is to choose wisely.

The food industry has been attempting to dupe us and destroy our health over the last 80-100 years. Prior to that time, food was grown by each family and cultivated for their own use or sold locally to other families. People were eating nutrient rich foods including vegetables, fruits, and grass-fed animal proteins. They also were involved in the work in harvesting the food which increased their activity level and their sun exposure naturally increasing their Vitamin D levels. As our country became more urban and less rural, the gradual assault and degradation of the quality of our food started. Large food companies and manufacturers started taking wholesome ingredients away and began to package the food in ways to maximize profits. The increased sugar and preservative content of the food significantly diminished the nutrition and increased the craving of this "junk." Their goals were to create addicts to their products similar to the way that drug dealers generate a market for their products. The food industry's version of heroin and cocaine however was a concoction that was as habitual and just as deadly. The craze has continued today to the point where over 60-70% of the U.S. population is considered overweight or obese. The government also chimed in to this façade by demonizing saturated fat and cholesterol per the work of Ancel Keys (dubbed the Father of Processed Foods) whom was a physiologist by trade whom performed fraudulent retrospective population studies. These studies completed in the 1950's were observational studies which suggests only an association and not randomized controlled trials which proves causation. Therefore, the power of the studies was low and the conclusions were incorrect. Yet, the false information that saturated fat and cholesterol cause heart disease and strokes continues today. The scary part is that it is not only the patients that believe these myths, but it is also many of the physicians. The truth is that processed sugar (carbohydrate), inflammation, hypertension, obesity, high triglycerides, insulin resistance, and hormone loss (estrogen/progesterone/testosterone/thyroid/DHEA) are the main culprits for these issues. Good luck finding or hearing this information unless you dig deep into the literature. The other byproduct of this fight against fat was the food pyramid put out by the USDA and endorsed by the American Heart Association in the 1970's. The recommendations of both groups focused on pushing carbohydrates and grains and limiting the intake of fats and protein. The end result was the explosion of weight gain in both adults and children thus propagating the obesity epidemic that persists today. This plays a major part in the increasing the use of healthcare and drugs which plays into the hand of the other players (insurance, hospitals, pharmaceutical, government) in this game. Unfortunately, this game is fixed against the participants and the patients become the Washington Generals (losers) to the healthcare titans/Harlem Globetrotters (winners).

The government has been a major part of the assault on American healthcare and the patients it claims to serve. As noted in the above paragraph, the government has been complicit in the dissemination of false and untrue information to the detriment of everybody involved. This sets an erroneous precedent(s) which takes decades to change in the minds of patients, physicians, administrators, policymakers, third party payers, etc. We again use "Bro Science or urban legend" to treat people as opposed to evidence-based medicine. Politicians and special interests also get involved to sway opinion and further confuse the situation. For example, the food industry pushes the falsehood that obesity is a patient problem caused by eating too many calories and exercising too little. Thus, they find a patsy for the obesity epidemic caused by their own products. To further enhance their bait and switch techniques, they then package 100 calorie snacks which are still nutrient poor and provide little in the way of changing the culture. Yet, they place the onus on the patient to control behavior and limit calories even though they are still garbage. The take home message is that 100 calories of Doritos are far different than 100 calories from walnuts or carrots. Don't be fooled into thinking all calories are the same and that the quality and content of the food holds no merit. Critically think and question information and dogma. I encourage you to do the same thing with myself and my information. If you don't like the answers and wish to go elsewhere, then at least you have made an informed decision.

The government is big business similar to the other entities that we have discussed.   The operation is run by politicians whom are primarily focused on satisfying their donors and getting re-elected. Thus, their goals (similar to the other players) do not align with your goals of excellent, affordable, efficient healthcare. They are focused on money, bigger budgets, special interests, and keeping their job. The government as well as the third-party payers want healthcare to remain expensive. Otherwise, their services would not be necessary. Per CDC statistics from 2016, healthcare spending reached $3.3 trillion which averaged to about $10,348 per person in the U.S. per year. Thus, the U.S. spent 17.9% of their GDP on healthcare and this total rises consistently each year. All of the villains (see above and below) give lip service to cutting costs and providing quality healthcare. In reality, their business is justified and flourishes via a sicker population and a higher cost for treatment. They all have little to no incentive to change unless they wish to eliminate jobs including their own, irritate their constituents, and aggravate their donors/special interests/villains. This issue thus becomes a campaign slogan for all parties involved and provides fodder for much debate. Gridlock however is ideal as no solutions are obtained and all the conspirators continue to get compensated in this American-style tragedy. The government has also been a major player in the deceptive practices of the food industry (food pyramid/obesity), the pharmaceutical industry (opioid crisis/pain as the 5th vital sign/no addictive properties related to opioid use), and the justice department (medical cannabis/federally illegal/schedule I drug although known medical uses). Looking into the future, there is no apparent cure or resolution for these deficiencies and concerns. The system at some point will collapse similar to the financial and housing sectors in the late 2000's. This is not an appetizing prospect and therefore you need to be proactive in looking for positive options like my practice for your healthcare needs.

Healthcare providers, including myself, have also been complicit in the healthcare conspiracy and thus a villain (think Darth Vader with heavy breathing). We too have placed our focus on treatments, procedures, surgeries, labs, imaging, and drugs that have a CPT code ultimately leading to payment as opposed to the best form of care. For example, joint pain in the spine (zygapophyseal joints or facet joints) is typically treated with intra-articular injections. If these fail, then radiofrequency lesioning (burning or frying) of the nerves innervating the joints is completed. This may help with the pain short-term but long-term causes problems as the muscles are denervated which serves to increase instability and pain. This procedure however has codes for both the injection procedure and the radiofrequency procedure and thus we receive remuneration. The better course of treatment would be to employ a regenerative medicine procedure such as prolotherapy or PRP to restore the integrity of the soft tissues and supporting structures and ultimately work with the anatomy instead of destroying it. The problem is that there is no code for this intervention and therefore an out of pocket expense for the patient. Due to the fact that we have some issue with asking for money, we cower and follow the path of least resistance and thus avoid a difficult conversation. We however then put the patient in harm's way because we have no backbone (pun intended again). Thus, insurance companies are consequently dictating care instead of the providers, and unfortunately, we allow it to occur hence becoming part of the problem. This thought process and mindset needs to change otherwise we are no better than the other villains. We, as a group, also tend to cling to old dogma and ineffectual treatments as propagated in medical school, residency, and continuing medical education courses (see prior chapters in relation to orthopedic and hormone treatments for examples). The mob mentality often exists where anything new is viewed as controversial or experimental at best and malpractice or quackery at worst. History has shown us that any idea that is transformative is oftentimes met with vehement resistance. Many topics in this book meet the definition of this statement. Change is difficult, but a necessary part of evolving and moving forward for both the patient (you) and the physician (me). Face it, the vast majority of patients are dissatisfied with their current level of care and the subsequent results. Join me in this venture and I'm certain that you will be enthusiastically gratified with your decision.

CHAPTER 16: THE HERO OF OUR DRAMA

The hero of this story and the real reason for writing this book is you (hence the title). As outlined in the prior chapters, the deck seems stacked against our hero. There are many impediments and negative influences impacting out hero's journey. There are also many different villains using their guile and evil powers to thwart our hero in his/her goal of obtaining optimal vitality and healthspan nirvana. The current healthcare environment is filled with landmines and obstacles. The main goal of most of those involved is to maximize dollars. Unfortunately, this flies in the face of maximizing your health as the sicker you are, the better it is for business. You, however, are smarter than those members of the Evil Empire (kudos to Rage Against the Machine), and you are a critical thinker and a rock star. You know what you want to treat and what you want to fix. Your goals and needs are thus unique to you, and therefore must be addressed in an independent and unconstrained manner. It is unethical and intrusive for so many other forces to have control over you and your health without placing your best interests at the forefront. It is now time for our hero (you) to escape the clutches of those trying to inflict harm and restrain you from reaching the pinnacle of life.

It is time for you to THRIVE instead of just survive. It is time for you to LIVE instead of just exist. It is time for you to KICK ASS instead of being beaten down. It is time to say I MATTER instead of I am invisible. It is time for you to be PROACTIVE instead of reactive. It is time for you to be part of the SOLUTION instead of continuing to be part of the problem. It is time for a new mindset where you start to

act like a HERO and not like a victim. It is time for you to
wrestle the wheel away and take CONTROL of the situation
instead of abdicating your power to others. It is time for you
to be viewed as a WHOLE PERSON instead of as a
diagnosis or a number. It is time that your problems are
SOLVED instead of managed with a litany of ineffective and
problematic medications. It is time for you to come out on
top. It is time for you to triumph. It is time for you to hit
the lottery. It is time for you to find the significant other of
your dreams. It is time for you to have mind-blowing sex. It
is time to stop hurting and malfunctioning. It is time to look
and feel like a million dollars. It is time for you to claim your
rightful place as the hero and conqueror. Don't be bashful
about it. Seize the day (Carpe Diem).

The transformation, however, must come from within
you, the hero. This approach and change cannot be forced
by others. It must mean something to you. You must have a
direction and a purpose. This may change with each visit,
procedure, exercise session, or treatment. You must
constantly evolve, strive, and diversify. This modus operandi
encourages growth as an individual and as a member of
society. The hero must ignore the naysayers and the critics.
These (the naysayers) are the same people that take few
chances yet belittle those that do. The hero must be willing
to trust their convictions and write their own story. The hero
must be willing to sacrifice something of value (like money
and time) to meet their goals. The hero must understand that
this is not accomplished in days, weeks, or months. It is
accomplished over a lifetime. It has to be something that you
want and covet, no matter the obstacles. You need to find
your calling and your muse. You need to use your anger and
drive as a gift for positive change. These are exactly the
people that I want to treat. These are the people that define
A NEW YOU!

CHAPTER 17: THE GUIDE

The evolution of YOU and your transformation is the sine qua non of the story. YOU are the main character, the one with the large star on your door. The one whom rides in limousines and is stalked by the paparazzi for pictures. YOU are the headliner. A good story however also needs a guide or guru to impart wisdom to the hero and allow them to reach their full potential. The guide is an integral part of the story, but he/she works behind the scene as an authority figure and as a rudder for the hero's proverbial ship. The guide must also empathize with the hero's dilemma(s), issue(s), or problem(s). This empathy typically comes from personal or professional experiences and creates a bond of trust. Donald Miller in his book Building a Story Brand noted that people (you as the hero) trust those who understand them. To hammer home this point as it relates to empathy, he quoted the quintessential guide, Oprah Winfrey. Oprah in her infinite wisdom explained the three things every human being wants are to be seen, heard, and understood. I therefore want to be that guide for YOU in your quest for health optimization focusing on the tenets of authority, empathy, and humility.

My role in this story is something that I covet and I embrace. I make a promise to deliver cutting edge and evidence-based treatments to help YOU in your journey and guide you toward health optimization. The focus will be on the body, the mind, and the spirit of the individual. There will be no judgement or prejudice on my part. You are the captain/king/hero of this epic tale, and I am the wizard behind the curtain keeping you on track and on the straight and narrow. Think of me as the Watson to your Sherlock Holmes. The Yoda to your Luke Skywalker. The Charles

Xavier to your Wolverine/Logan. The Q to your James Bond. The Mickie to your Rocky Balboa. The Steve Trevor to your Wonder Woman. I think you get the picture as to the relationship and the potential for unlimited benefit. Similar to the aforementioned examples, the essential link between all of them is the fact that they were life-long and longstanding relationships. Thus, I want to impart the reality that our interaction will need to be long term to meet your goals. Understand that goals will change and these issues will be a moving target. At times, it is like a giant game of whack a mole. The beauty of our relationship will be that all of our treatments and interventions are intertwined. I will be addressing your issues from head to toe with little in the way of compartmentalization. There will be no deferral as to your concerns or issues. If I am unable to solve your problem, then I will have a network of experts that our office will help you navigate to address your specific issue. At times, I will be the end point and the solution. At other times, I will act as a quarterback of a football team or the conductor of a symphony in coordinating your care and treatment.

My job is thus to use my professional experiences, personal experiences, and knowledge to formulate an individual plan of attack to cure your ailments. I, therefore, provide a pathway to resolve your issue(s) using the options outlined in this book along with many others. Medicine and technology change so quickly that new treatments and interventions are approved and implemented thus adding to my armamentarium. This benefits you as a patient and ultimately provides more targeted and less invasive means to positively affect your health. This inclusive and exclusive course of action should provide clarity for you as the patient such that the fear and concern is removed from the equation, thus we can focus on the process of healing and transforming.

A clear plan with clarity provides a blueprint for you to tackle the difficulties that confront your life and health on a daily basis. While it is important to read, research, and review potential options for treatment for your specific health issues; you need a medical guru or savant like myself to pare down the information and coordinate a focused unique plan to address your issues. Therefore, I am the conduit between you and the medical world to formulate your cure plan. I am your wizard. I am your shaman. I am your soothsayer. I am your authority. I am your master. I work for you and not the reverse. The work that I do for you should make the course of action easy to implement and follow without confusing jargon. Your work primarily should focus on getting better and reaching your goals. As an example, I will use IKEA. While it may be cheaper and satisfying to buy raw materials and fabricate a bookshelf or table on your own, there is a trade-off. You give up time and energy. There is also the potential frustration factor related to poor directions and missing pieces which may negatively affect your health by raising your stress and cortisol levels. The alternative option includes buying a fabricated table or bookshelf or hiring somebody to build the one you purchase from IKEA. While the cost may be more, you free up time for your own activities and limit stress all while achieving your goal of a new bookshelf or table. I want to be the fabricator and builder of A NEW YOU. We are all busy and limited with our time. I want you focused on the process and the journey toward vitality as opposed to the minutia. The clarity of the plan will be my promise and the easy part for you, the hard part will be the blood, sweat, and tears involved in obtaining the goal or goals.

CHAPTER 18: SEXUAL HEALTH and FUNCTION / DYSFUNCTION; REMOVING THE TABOOS and STIGMAS

Sexuality and sexual health are topics that are typically ignored in the vast majority of healthcare evaluations. The reasons for this omission are numerous. These include embarrassment on the part of the patient and physician, societal taboos and stigmas with the topic, religious beliefs, labels, ridicule, and privacy concerns. None of these excuses however hold water and should not deter the hero from seeking information and treatment on this matter. Sex is one of our most intimate experiences and primal activities. It solidifies a relationship and provides another means to share joy, improve communication, and explore desires and fantasies. From a clinical standpoint, sex has also been shown to lengthen life, lower the risk of cardiovascular disease, augment immune system function, reduce depression and stress, improve brain function, positively affect pain, correct sleep dysfunction, fight prostate cancer, improve aesthetics/skin integrity, and add happiness and meaning to life. From a human standpoint, people whom are sexually active tend to be more social and socially inclusive. People whom are connected tend to live healthier and more vibrant lives.

Female sexual dysfunction may affect a woman at any age. The reasons are multiple and varied. Each of them may have a deleterious effect on the quality of life and vitality. We will delve into a few of the most common issues to provide some examples. The first and potentially most common are hormone-related changes. These may occur at or near menopause but may be altered at any time during the lifespan. The hormones affected include estrogen, progesterone, testosterone, thyroid, DHEA, Vitamin D, and human growth hormone. These topics have been discussed in more detail in other portions of the book, but needless to say their effect on sexual function can be profound. Deficiency of these substances may have a negative effect on energy, sexual arousal, libido, performance, vaginal lubrication, and orgasm. The second set of problems revolve around orthopedic dysfunction and fitness deficits such as physical strength, stamina, joint health, and bone health may also have a deleterious effect. These problems may seem to fall outside the realm of sexual activity and function. Musculoskeletal issues however may affect the number of sexual positions and thus variety. It also may affect enjoyment due to pain, range of motion deficits, the possibility for fracture, and the inability to orgasm due to myofascial dysfunction/pelvic floor weakness. The third set of problems are metabolic disorders such as diabetes mellitus, obesity, metabolic syndrome, and hyperthyroidism. The fourth set of problems are cardiac-related and include hypertension, coronary artery disease, myocardial infarction (heart attack), arrhythmias, congestive heart failure, and bypass grafting. The fifth set of issues are neurological including stroke, multiple sclerosis, vascular dementia, Alzheimer's disease, spinal cord injury, and peripheral nerve injury. The sixth category include cancers of the breast, uterus, ovaries, vagina, brain, and skin. The seventh set are lifetime achievement awards such as urinary incontinence, vaginal atrophy and dryness, diminished sensation in the clitoris/sexual organs, anorgasmia, decreased nipple sensation, and limited engagement/desire (from the brain which is the most important sex organ). The next group would encompass negative side effects of agents/interventions or mindbody alterations. This list may include medications like antidepressants and anti-anxiety agents, treatments like chemotherapy and radiation, surgeries like cardiac bypass and hysterectomy, disfiguring procedures such as a mastectomy or a colostomy, trauma such as rape and sexual assault, and mental health problems such as bipolar disorder and depression. The last group would involve idiopathic processes such as interstitial cystitis and lichen sclerosus which can be quite debilitating and life altering. The treatments for these issues are scant and primarily involve addressing the symptoms as opposed to the root cause of the problem. Women with these issues are oftentimes miserable due to the pain and discomfort which causes isolation and marital/relationship problems.

As we see from the information contained in the above paragraph, there is not a health issue or problem that does not affect sexual function. Yet, rarely are these issues discussed, addressed, treated, or prevented in any fashion by the medical community. I therefore feel that this is an area that is ripe for engagement as a way to treat a woman or a man as a whole person as opposed to a disease or a symptom. The beauty of managing sexual problems is the deeper connection that may occur with the patient and their significant other. If we are able to solve these dysfunctions or deficiencies, then the trust between us multiplies exponentially thus solidifying our professional relationship with the goal of maximizing your health. The transformation includes many of the treatments that have been touched on in other parts of the book including exercise, diet and nutrition, supplements, bio-identical hormone replacement, and orthopedic/musculoskeletal interventions. The new exciting part of sexual health medicine includes the use of platelet rich plasma (PRP) for injection into the clitoral area and the urethral/vagina interface. This procedure is called an O-shot or an Orgasm shot. This procedure was popularized and trademarked by Dr. Charles Runels in Fairhope, Alabama. I recently attended his course which was an outstanding combination of clinical aesthetic and sexual medicine as well as marketing and promoting. I would highly recommend this course to any provider whom is looking to help more patients and provide services that are sorely lacking in our society. The O-shot is an outpatient procedure that benefits women with orgasm problems, vaginal lubrication and atrophy problems, bladder incontinence, lichen sclerosus, interstitial cystitis, postsurgical pain/episiotomy scars, and dyspareunia/painful sex. The procedure takes 5-10 minutes to perform and works to rejuvenate and restore tissue by increasing blood flow, recruiting growth factors, stimulating fibroblasts and stem cells, and changing the integrity/environment of the tissue. These actions encourage a rebirth and a revascularization of the tissue which can be life changing. These effects may be augmented with vaginal rejuvenation procedures which include radiofrequency lesioning and laser. The PRP may also be used for injection in the breast for augmentation, the hair for growth, and the face with Juvaderm for rejuvenation (Vampire Facelift). These procedures work similarly to the O-shot and orthopedic interventions to help with aesthetics, function, and restoration.

Male sexual dysfunction also is intertwined with many health issues and disease processes. I will not repeat the list from the above paragraph as there is significant crossover, but I will add a few male specific problems that may cause problems. These include hypogonadism/andropause/low testosterone, thyroid dysfunction, prostate cancer/surgery, diabetes mellitus, DHEA deficiency, stress, mental health issues, medication side effects (beta blockers like Propranolol, hair restoration drugs like Propecia, benign prostatic hypertrophy drugs like Avodart, and antidepressants like Celexa), surgeries (like cardiac bypass grafting, colon resection for cancer, and brain surgery/craniotomy), obesity, metabolic syndrome (diabetes mellitus/hypertension/high triglycerides/increased visceral fat), chronic infection (like prostatitis), lichen sclerosus, and a physical impairment/disability. This is not an exhaustive list but provides context to men as possible issues that may afflict them throughout their lifespan and alter their sexual function and sense of masculinity. For men, there is a PRP injection called the P-shot or Priapus shot which involves four injections along the length of the penis and one injection into the head of the penis. The goals are similar to those outlined under the O-shot to improve blood flow, release growth factors, recruit fibroblasts/stem cells, and improve the environment for rejuvenation and restoration. The procedure takes 5-10 minutes to perform and is typically followed by use of a penis pump for 5-10 minutes twice a day at -10 mm of Hg. The procedure may also be accentuated by electrical stimulation with the most common device used called a Gaines wave. This procedure is indicated for men with erectile dysfunction, lichen sclerosus, Peyronie's disease (curve of the penis due to scarring), and postoperative problems following prostate surgery. I have had the procedure done and there is minimal discomfort after topical anesthesia and/or soft tissue anesthesia via lidocaine. These interventions may be used in addition to or in place of erectile dysfunction drugs like Viagra, Cialis, and Levitra. PRP may also be used/injected in men to help with hair growth and facial aesthetics (Vampire Facelift).

 As we have learned, sexual health issues have real causes and real consequences in life. When difficulties occur, it can affect mood, self-esteem, happiness, and vitality. Addressing these issues with a medical professional and solving the dysfunction may help to save relationships and marriages thus reducing the possibility for divorce and infidelity. Treatment may also improve the bond between partners such that love is rekindled and new territories and activities are explored. It thus becomes imperative for the physician or healthcare provider to be proactive and initiate a conversation on the topic. It is also important to educate our patients via talks, videos, books, pamphlets, and emails. Most mainstream physicians know very little about this information and will likely downplay the benefits due to ignorance or bias. It is therefore incumbent upon the small minority of enlightened providers to spread the word via both a grassroots and social media approach to directly disseminate and inform the public. This ultimately maximizes a positive outcome for all involved and provides personal satisfaction for the patient and professional joy for the provider. The take home message and call to action for you as the patient is twofold. One, take personal responsibility for your health including your sexual function. Two, evolution and change as a patient involves movement out of your comfort zone and into unchartered territory. Fear not asking questions and broaching difficult topics. Understand that I am not a mind reader. If you fail to address an issue because you are embarrassed or fearful, then you have nobody to blame but the person looking at you in the mirror. There will be no judgment, just understanding and compassion along with a clear plan formulated for resolution and cure as opposed to symptom management. Trust me as I truly trust you due to the fact that you have graciously chosen me to heal you.

I would be remiss in discussing this topic if I failed to address the issues with sexual identity and sexual attitudes. Whether you identify as homosexual, bisexual, transsexual, asexual, hypersexual, or a sexual "deviant," the emotional and psychological toll of these identities or labels can be

overwhelming. Adolescents, teens, and adults whom fall
outside of the societal "norms" of heterosexuality are
oftentimes ridiculed, ignored, ostracized, and isolated. The
suicide rate for all members of our society has increased over
the last 5-10 years, but this group of individuals is particularly
hard hit due to the struggle internally and the turmoil from
others externally. This negativity may emanate from multiple
sources which may include parents, siblings, friends,
significant others, teachers, healthcare professionals, and total
strangers. Acknowledgment, acceptance, education, and
support are both anticipated and expected by those wishing
to share their singular stories. When this narrative is met with
resistance from those whom they care about and respect, the
effects may be devastating both in the short and long term.
Medical care for these unique and exceptional individuals may
also suffer due to fear and uneasiness from the patient and
inherent biases and judgmental behaviors from the providers.
No matter how you identify yourself, you too are the hero of
your story in need of a guide in striving for optimal health. I
promise to be that guru for you and commit to treat you as
you would wish to be treated. The focus is on you and your
needs, not those of anybody else involved in your life and
care. I/we will focus on what will make you happy and
content, thus restoring and rejuvenating A NEW YOU.

CHAPTER 19: EXERCISE and HEALTH

Exercise is the cornerstone and provides the foundation for implementation of a treatment regimen for your ailments and deficiencies. This includes orthopedic abnormalities, functional weakness and dysfunction, hormone imbalances, sexual health dysfunctions, and aesthetic problems. Exercise provides a pathway for sustaining overall health, wellness, and vitality. As humans, we were born to move and thus activity must be part of the equation. Regular activity serves to improve blood flow, lung capacity, strength, flexibility, aerobic fitness, anaerobic threshold, visceral fat levels, inflammation, and insulin resistance. The benefits include a decreased risk of heart disease, stroke, hypertension, cancer, anxiety, depression, and memory loss. For example, a Duke University study from 1999 assessed the effect of exercise on depression. The participants performed 45 minutes of aerobic exercise three times per week. The results from the study showed that the exercise group responded better to depression than those patients whom were treated with Zoloft. Exercise is low cost, readily available, beneficial, risk averse, and mood enhancing. This intervention should be the first prescription that medical providers should order no matter the problem. There is essentially no downside with this form of treatment with tons of upside. Return on investment is high with minimal chance for loss.

Exercise is regenerative and restorative medicine. Regular activity and exercise may extend the lifespan by at least five years. Exercise improves the number of mitochondria in the cells. Mitochondria are the powerhouses of the cell and provide energy via respiration. The higher the number of mitochondria, the better the health of the cell, tissue, organ, and individual. Progressive weight training over six months (including heavy total body movements like the squat and deadlift) has been shown to reverse aging in patients via an increase in mitochondrial density as well as an increase in telomere length. Moderate exercise slows the aging of cells and protects telomeres. Telomeres are located at the end of chromosomes and progressively shorten with each cell division. These typically shorten with age and ultimately cause senescence or cell death. Senescent cells are problematic as they are pro-inflammatory and may affect other parts of the body and negatively affect the health of the individual. Accelerated telomere shortening is associated with chronic health problems including diabetes mellitus, congestive heart failure, coronary artery disease, myocardial infarction, cancer, and osteoporosis. In the elderly, it helps to predict mortality. Smoking cessation, weight loss, exercise, and positive dietary changes all improve telomere length, health, and lifespan. All of these interventions will be used via a comprehensive approach to help enhance you and your health.

There are many forms of activity and exercise combinations that may be used in a comprehensive and all-encompassing program. The primary focus in my opinion however must revolve around strength training. Humans begin to lose muscle mass and strength starting in their 30's to the tune of 1-2% per year. This tends to accelerate as we age to the point where significant sarcopenia (muscle wasting) may occur. Resistance training halts muscle atrophy and increases skeletal muscle mass. This effect is further enhanced via supplementation with testosterone, DHEA, and growth hormone. Strength and resistance training also replace slow twitch type I fibers with fast twitch type II fibers. Stimulation and recruitment of type II fibers via strength training are better than cardiovascular and aerobic fitness exercise for fat loss and weight control. The benefits are thus endless and include improvements for muscle, bone, cardiovascular, neurological, skin, metabolic, and hormonal health. This intervention and its multiple iterations have four major goals: limit impairment, guard against disability, limit falls and fractures, and maintain independence. Strength training checks all of the boxes on that list and many others. In combination with hormone replacement, supplementation, and regenerative orthopedic interventions; resistance training is a major component of a healthy lifestyle and provides a significant boost in longevity and lifespan. Alternative exercises used as adjuncts to strength training include Pilates, yoga, Zumba, walking, running, swimming, cycling, tennis golf, etc. The take home point is that movement and activity must become an integral part of the health equation and failure to incorporate them into your regimen sets you up for failure.

A study from Penn State University looked at the effect of resistance training on the health of older adults. The study group exercised via strength and resistance training two times per week. The results were striking for the exercise group as compared to the control group. They had 46% lower odds of all cause death and 41% lower odds of cardiac death. They also had 19% lower odds of dying from cancer. Thus, exercise is medicine and a form of anti-aging and longevity management.

Heat stress including sauna training has also been shown to be a treatment for maintaining muscle mass via the release of heat shock proteins and growth hormone. The patient must remain in the environment for at least 15-30 minutes to realize the positive response. In rat studies, heat increased muscle regrowth by about 30%. The addition of heat as a treatment option has been shown to increase longevity and may be used as an adjunctive tool for maintenance and growth of muscle. When heat treatment was combined with exercise like yoga, push-ups, or body weight squats in the sauna environment, the muscle growth was further accentuated. The benefits of sweating may also be profound from a health standpoint in removing toxins including heavy metals from the body such as arsenic, cadmium, lead, and mercury. This activity is an easy and low-cost detoxification process which serves to further optimize and improve health.

The goal of exercise therefore is to maximize function via gains in strength, muscle mass, mitochondrial density, telomere length, and hormonal stimulation. It decreases visceral fat and ultimately improves insulin resistance. This serves to limit insulin surges which typically place the body in a catabolic (breakdown) state. This intervention also assists in decreasing inflammatory processes in the body which further improves overall health and wellness. Diffuse inflammation is a precursor for chronic disease and substandard health, and simple interventions like exercise are integral in combating the deleterious effects of this condition. Exercise also serves to improve and elevate mood, increase blood flow and cardiac output, decrease vascular resistance and blood pressure, and maximize lung function. Sexual function also improves via improvements in strength, flexibility, and aerobic stamina. In my opinion, there are only advantages and positive outcomes with the addition of exercise and performance training. This energy pervades this book and ties in nicely with the ultimate goal of improving your health. I encourage you to embrace it and find your niche activity/activities thus allowing you to reach your maximum potential.

CHAPTER 20: THE PACT

We now have come to the point in time where we need to discuss the etiquette as it relates to our interaction and alliance. The doctor-patient relationship in my opinion is based on trust and truth. These two tenets are the primary basis for delivering on the promise to heal, fix, and transform you.

The definition of truth via Webster's dictionary is conformity with fact or reality. In addition, truth also means accuracy, honesty and integrity. I believe that all of these words and phrases apply as a foundation for our process and journey. We must both understand that truth works reciprocally. We both must be willing to be brutally honest with each other if we want to affect the change and transformation that you crave. This means that you get what you give. I am unable to guide and treat you effectively unless we take a deep dive into challenging and difficult topics. For example, sexual dysfunction may be the result of mental or physical abuse by a family member, significant other, or a trusted source (such as a teacher or clergy person). Without the truth and this key piece of information, we may fail to adequately fix your problem due to a limited focus on the root cause of the problem. To quote Lana Lang, "Life is about change. Sometimes it's painful. Sometimes it's beautiful. But most of the time it is both."

Trust thus is the outgrowth of sharing the truth and forging a relationship based on mutual respect and goals. Webster's definition of trust is confident expectation of something; reliance on the integrity, strength, ability, and surety of a person or thing; confidence; hope. I believe in all of these words and statements, and with that comes tremendous responsibility. You must understand and trust that I have your back, and I have your best interests at heart. Trust that I am your life preserver and I will never waver from my role as your guide. I, too, must trust you to become fully engaged in our program and execute the plan as outlined. The relationship is like a football coach and a quarterback or like a teacher and student. Yet, the topics discussed will be more in-depth and private than any of those relationships may be. Our discussions may be more intimate than those you have with a spouse, friend, or family member. All of this entails and is built upon trust. You have made an appointment with our facility and ultimately shown that you trust me and my team to help you. You have shown an interest and a desire to transform and change for the positive. Socrates opined, "The secret of change is to focus all of your energy, not on fighting the old, but on building the new." This personal development requires truth and trust. This requires three commitments. The first, you must be truthful and trustworthy with yourself. The second, you must be truthful and trustworthy with me. The third, I must be truthful and trustworthy with you, your journey, and our process.

We, therefore, will seal our relationship with a written pact or contract. This document binds us and will be specific to your needs and not a generic template or arrangement. This serves as a framework to outline our goals, benchmarks, and commitments to one another. This record also makes us accountable to one another and chronicles our promise to one another. It makes us beholden to the process and also establishes boundaries. It also confirms and explains my plan to make you uncomfortable. My job is to push you out of your comfort zone and get you to think outside of the box. This action will provide a different perspective and encourage critical thinking. For you to move forward, we may have to tackle painful and difficult subjects which may cause turmoil or irritation. We may need to break you down and take a few steps backwards prior to transforming, rebuilding, and optimizing you. This exercise may be a necessary evil to remove the clutter and fear from your life such that we may help you to progress. Arnold Bennett noted, "Any change, even a change for the better, is always accompanied by drawbacks and discomforts." I encourage you to embrace the process and the journey thus freeing your mind to improve your wellness. My passion and energy will be focused on providing knowledge and destroying the myths and incorrect information that pervades medicine and fitness. Evidence-based literature, techniques, treatments, and processes will be employed in a concerted effort to heal you. The reason you sought my help likely stems from the fact that you were not happy with the level of care you were receiving. If you are honest with yourself in self-reflection, you may also have noted that your attitude and thoughts may have also limited your response to management. Sometimes, we are our own worst enemies as our entrenched thoughts restrict our ability to evolve. Max Dupree stated, "We cannot become what we want by remaining what we are." To further emphasize this point, Albert Einstein cited, "The world as we have created it is a process of your thinking. It cannot be changed without changing our thinking." Last quote and this comes from me and thus a Meighen special, "If you are not part of the solution, then you are part of the problem."

CHAPTER 21: THE RULES

I have now weaved a tale as it relates to providing quality healthcare and improving the quality of life of you, the individual patient and hero. I have described in detail the main approaches I will employ as it pertains to achieving these goals. My promise and pledge to forge A NEW YOU. There however is one final step and process to discuss prior to determining if we are a good fit to work together. I call these the Do's and Don'ts. I have certain beliefs as it relates to common courtesy and decency in any type or relationship, but especially with a patient. I want us to be on the same page from the beginning with no innuendo or hidden agenda. I am entering this information into my book, website, social media, etc. to provide clarity and transparency as to my expectations. Thus, there are no mixed messages or hidden items. Our values and culture will be posted and palpable through our actions and interactions with our patients/clients. These values are as follows: humility, commitment, accountability and zeal. I will demand of myself and my staff that we live up these words and exceed our promise to you and over-deliver.

I therefore will now outline the things I want from an ideal patient/client to maximize the experience both for you as the hero and myself as the guide. I left conventional medicine and sick care due to the constraints of the process and the limited control I had over all aspects of my life. This new iteration will ultimately serve to make this a positive experience for all players involved including myself and allow me to disengage from adversarial and negative interactions.

With this as a backdrop, here are the list of Do's for a positive relationship and interaction:

1. Enter with an open mind and be willing to think critically.
2. Be open, honest, truthful, and unhindered in your responses and answers. Understand I am not a mind reader and I cannot help you fix a problem without knowledge of said problem
3. Understand that change and transformation occur over time and that progress may be slow. Therefore, this requires a long-term commitment. Your problem will not be fixed in 1-2 visits or with a simple procedure.
4. Check your ego at the door and enter with humility
5. Intimate topics including sexual activity, pleasure, masturbation, sexual dysfunction, desires, and goals will be discussed in detail. Understand that the intention is to fix a problem and rejuvenate your relationship with yourself and your significant other. The aim is to gather information and not to pry. There are no judgments here, only solutions.
6. Complete all intake paperwork online prior to your appointment time. This eliminates inefficiency and allows me to focus on you. Failure to adhere to this rule will require your appointment to be rescheduled. This is non-negotiable.
7. Show up on time. Tardiness and excuses will not be accepted for any reason. Your appointment will thus be rescheduled if this should occur. This again is non-negotiable.
8. Provide a list with dosages of all of your medications. Provide a list of your drug allergies.
9. Enter with a calm polite demeanor and treat everybody involved in your care with respect and civility. Treat people as you would like to be treated.

10. Obtain all pertinent medical records, films, reports, labs, etc. and provide them to our office for review prior to your appointment. This improves efficiency and allows us to formulate a preliminary plan prior to your evaluation.

11. Understand that I have your best interests at heart and I will not put you in harm's way. This does not, however, mean that the treatments are risk free and without potential side effects. It does mean that the plan will be individualized to your needs and implemented to maximize a positive outcome and minimize a negative one.

12. Implement the plan as discussed and outlined in our interactions. If you fail to follow the plan, then it is difficult to make appropriate changes and adjustments as the data is now flawed. If this should occur, then I will dissolve the contract and recommend that you see another provider. Noncompliance shows me a lack of trust and respect which will poison our relationship and lead to failure.

13. Listen, learn, research, and ACT.

14. Pay your bill in full when requested to do so by our office. You will be provided with three options. Cash, credit, or Care Credit. There are no payment plans or balances. You may make monthly payments but no treatment will be rendered until you are paid in full. This rule again is non-negotiable.

15. Please provide a testimonial, positive review, and/or a social media post if you enjoyed our services and wish to recommend us to others.

16. Provide a positive vibe and energy as this transformation process into A NEW YOU evolves. Understand that happiness is infectious.

This will be the list of Don'ts that will negatively affect our relationship and be a cause for expulsion from the park (insert name of your favorite amusement park here):

1. Showing up late
2. Failing to complete your paperwork and/or homework prior to presentation to the office
3. Sexually harassing or verbally abusing myself or any member of the staff
4. Requesting refills of opioid pain relievers, benzodiazepines, anxiolytics, or sleep aids. Our goal is to eliminate the need for a number of your medications and resolve the epidemic of polypharmacy.
5. Saying phrases such as I can't, I won't, I don't have time, or I'm too busy. Using any other negative language. What you are really saying is that my health is not my priority. If this is the case, then I recommend you find another provider.
6. Bigotry, racism, sexism, and misogyny will not be accepted or tolerated.
7. An unwillingness to engage in exercise or physical activity
8. A discussion of politics, religion, law, etc. that serves to cause divisiveness and emotions. These topics however may be discussed if they are germane to your problem and would provide context as a way to solve it.
9. Bring a firearm or weapon into the clinic.
10. Film or record anything in the clinic.
11. Failure to provide a credit card or bank card prior to the first appointment.
12. Making up your own rules.
13. Forging documents or stealing items including prescription pads.

14. Requesting that I contact or justify my treatment plans with your primary MD or any of your other providers. This again connotates a lack of trust and buy-in on your part thus eliminating our ability to work together.

15. Unwarranted negative reviews and antagonistic self-serving posts on social media that have the effect of sabotaging our relationship. Warranted concerns and criticisms are always encouraged and welcomed as a way to help us learn, grow, and transform as a clinic. I encourage a free dialogue and interaction to make this the best experience possible.

16. Failure to take responsibility for your own lot in life and blaming others for your current situation. I believe in the Extreme Ownership model as put forth by Jocko Willink in the book of the same title. You must own all of your actions (good and bad) and the results. Responsibility and owning success and failure makes a good leader/physician/patient/CEO. Blaming others for your shortcomings and failures results in negativity and portends weak character. Be the former (extreme owner) and not the latter (blameless weakling).

17. Making excuses and showing an unwillingness to change or evolve. Great people understand their flaws and limitations and try to correct them. Weak people ignore limitations and use them as obstacles to remain fixed in their current position. Be the change that you want to see in the mirror, on the scale, in the gym, in the bedroom, and in life.

18. Limited ambition to grow and improve with the feeling that you have made it. I have leaders in my own Mastermind and Advisor groups whom are quite successful and multimillionaires running companies

and medical practices. The reason that they join these groups is their constant search for knowledge and a quest to improve. We are all day to day. The goal is to be your best that day and to continually repeat the process moving forward.

CHAPTER 22: A CALL TO ACTION

I have now discussed the major topics and provided the information that I wished to portray as it relates to a paradigm shift in healthcare delivery and wellness. I have made my case that our current system is broken and focused more on profits as opposed to the individual patient. I have outlined my three-pronged approach for management including non-operative regenerative orthopedic medicine, bio-identical hormone replacement and functional medicine, and sexual and aesthetic medicine. I have expressed my passion and desire to optimize health in each individual patient whom seeks an alternative to the tried and true systems that have failed them. I want to attract people whom are hungry for something new and exciting. I want grinders whom fail to accept average and strive for excellence in all facets of their life. I want people whom are willing to give the middle finger to the same old same old, conformity, and stagnation. I want people whom want to act. If not now, then when? To quote Oscar Wilde, "To live is the rarest thing in the world. Most people exist. That is all." Do you see yourself in this quote? Are you just surviving or really thriving? What are you willing to change to meet these goals? It is time. Are you ready? Are you prepared to act?

www.EmpoweredWellnessNC.com

I thus will provide a call to action to the hero (you) such that you reclaim your overall health, vitality, and zest for life.

ATTENTION:

I believe that the current medical delivery system is broken. Physicians and patients are fed up and unhappy with the limitations and depersonalized delivery of the services rendered. Quality time spent with patients has significantly decreased due to the intrusive and time-consuming nature of electronic medical records and the reduced remuneration from payers (resulting in the need to see more patients in a compressed and finite time frame). Individual patients and the population as a whole have become sicker with each passing year despite spending nearly 20% of the GDP on healthcare in the United States.

More than 50% of physicians are burned out and looking for alternative careers within medicine. Others are leaving medicine totally and looking for alternative careers. A recent report from the Association of American Medical Colleges (printed by NBC News) projects a shortage of between 42,600 and 121,300 by 2030. This physician shortage will further exacerbate the problem ultimately overloading the system and decreasing satisfaction for all of those involved. Physicians have become highly paid scribes entering useless data into a document that wastes time, increases the cost of care, and fails to improve delivery of treatment. It serves as a tool (via the IT industry and third-party payers) to create obstacles that must be traversed in order to treat and manage problems. Even then, care is oftentimes denied due to cost, arbitrary rules, and special interest groups. This removes the doctor from their love, passion, and goal of caring for patients and optimizing health outcomes. Patient care has thus become secondary or tertiary in the healthcare system behind documentation and profit maximization. The system has lost its focus as to the primary reason for its very existence: To care for patients.

Are you interested in individual and personalized treatment and transformation without intrusion from insurance companies, the pharmaceutical industry, the food corporations, large healthcare conglomerates, and the government? Do you desire and crave a new perspective from a physician whom uses evidence-based treatments to restore, regenerate, and rejuvenate your health and vitality? Or do you wish to maintain a relationship with physicians whom peddle the party line of the sick care model with the primary goal of <u>M</u>aintaining <u>D</u>isease? Do you want **A NEW YOU**?

Do you want a non-conventional and fresh approach to healthcare and wellness that elevates you, the patient, as the focal point? Do you desire a practice that focuses on fitness and exercise, hormone optimization, regenerative non-operative orthopedic medicine (using you to heal you), sexual health evaluation and treatments, aesthetics, and overall function? Do you want to change? Do you want **A NEW YOU**? If so, then I implore you to take action and contact us at **EMPOWERED WELLNESS OF NORTH CAROLINA** to schedule a consult.

About Michael Meighen

Dr. Michael Meighen is a musculoskeletal specialist whom primarily focuses on conservative and non- operative measures to help patients with function and pain control. The main focus of his treatment plan centers around exercise and functional restoration; but he also incorporates adjunctive options including manipulation, injection therapy, oral medication, acupuncture, massage, etc. to meet the desired

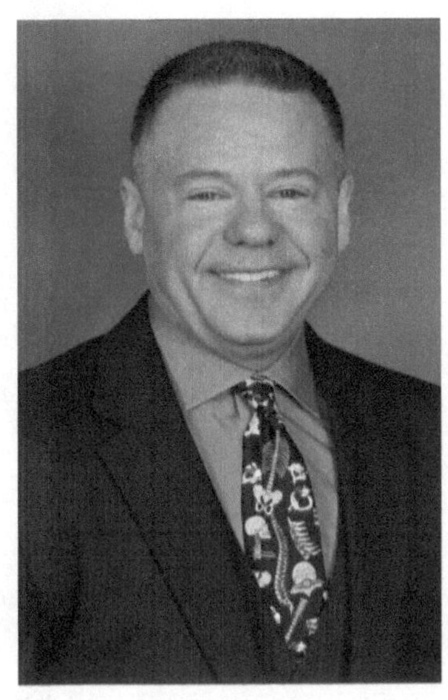

goal. He feels as though the patient has to be an active participant in care and part of the solution for management.

Dr. Meighen grew up in Northeast Ohio which instilled in him a strong work ethic and focus. This region of the country also fostered a love and passion for exercise and health. He graduated from the University of Toledo with a BA in Biology. During this time, he spent time studying in Manchester, England which provided him insight into an alternative culture and health care system. He then enrolled at the University of Akron where he completed a year of Master's studies in Sports Medicine. He next graduated from the University of Cincinnati with his medical degree with a goal of working in the orthopedic and musculoskeletal field. To meet these ends, he completed his Physical Medicine and Rehabilitation residency at Carolinas Medical Center/Charlotte Rehabilitation in Charlotte, NC. He then moved on to the University of Florida where he completed a fellowship in sports, spine, and occupational rehabilitation medicine under the tutelage of James Atchison, D.O.

Dr. Meighen in the past has worked for a large multispecialty orthopedic group in North Carolina which provided him with valuable insights into the management of musculoskeletal problems. He has extensive experience and knowledge in the treatment of spine, joint, and soft tissue abnormalities. He has a passion for the field, and he uses a multimodal approach employing new and leading-edge techniques to solve pain problems. He is well versed in the following interventions to help diagnose and treat musculoskeletal disorders: fluoroscopically guided spine and joint procedures, diagnostic and interventional ultrasound, electrodiagnostics (EMG/NCS), osteopathic manipulation, and regenerative procedures including prolotherapy, platelet rich plasma (PRP), and stem cells. He also has specialized training in bio-identical hormone replacement and wellness.

Michael was voted one of Charlotte Business Journal's Best Physicians in 2012-2014, he is Board Certified in Physical Medicine and Rehabilitation and Pain Medicine, Advanced Bioidentical Hormone Replacement Certification from WorldLink Medical.

He can be reached at www.EmpoweredWellnessNC.com or contacted directly at MeighenMD@gmail.com.

Book Michael Meighen to Speak

Book Michael Meighen as Your Keynote Speaker and You're Guaranteed to Make Your Event Inspirational, Motivational, Highly Entertaining, and Unforgettable!

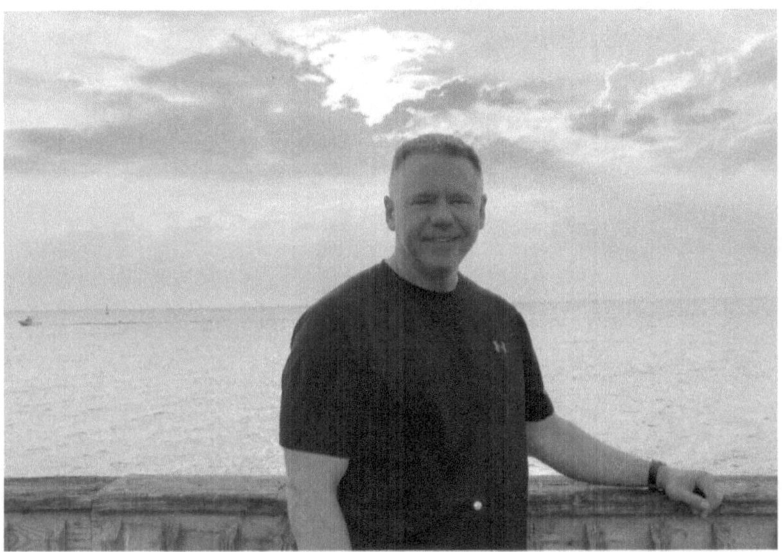

For over two decades, Dr. Michael Meighen has treated and healed more than 25,000 patients in his practice.

Today, he's transforming health care by using and implementing the latest, cutting-edge treatments to increase his patients' energy, vitality, movement, sense of well-being impact, income *and quality of life*.

Now he's taking his message and systems to people and organizations that want to experience change, be inspired and achieve high-performance both in business and life by improving their health.

His #1 Bestselling Book, "A New You: Using the Body's Regenerative and Restorative Healing Powers to

Optimize Orthopedic, Hormonal and Sexual Health Function" provided the backdrop of his breakthrough work and treatment systems.

His unique style inspires, empowers, and entertains audiences while giving them the tools and strategies you need to bring hope, awareness and transformation into businesses and organizations that want their employees and members to experience the highest level of performance and capabilities.

For more info and to book Dr. Meighen for your next event, send an email to MeighenMD@gmail.com.